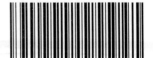

Table of Contents

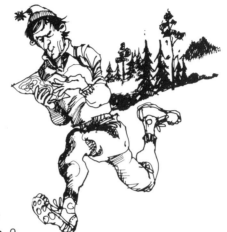

Table of Contents

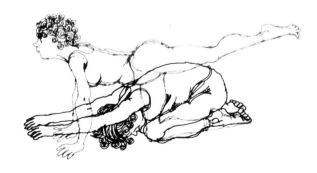

HEALTH AND FITNESS

by
P.O. Åstrand, M.D.

Department of Physiology
Gymastik-ock Idrottshogskolan
Stockholm, Sweden

Barron's/Woodbury, New York

The original text was published by the
Skandia Insurance Company Ltd.,
Stockholm, and the Swedish Information
Services, with drawings by Claes Folcker. It is
adapted by permission of the copyright
holders.

© Copyright 1977 by Barron's Educational Series, Inc.

All inquiries should be addressed to:
Barron's Educational Series, Inc.
113 Crossways Park Drive
Woodbury, New York 11797

Library of Congress Catalog Card No. 76-54305

International Standard Book No. 0-8120-0775-1

Library of Congress Cataloging in Publication Data
Astrand, Per Olof
  Health and fitness.
  Bibliography: p.
  1. Exercise. 2. Physical fitness. I. Title.
[DNLM: 1. Physical fitness — Popular works.
2. Gymnastics. 3. Hygiene—Popular works.
QT255 A859k]
RA781.A78   1976   613.7'1   76-54305
ISBN 0-8120-0775-1

PRINTED IN THE UNITED STATES OF AMERICA

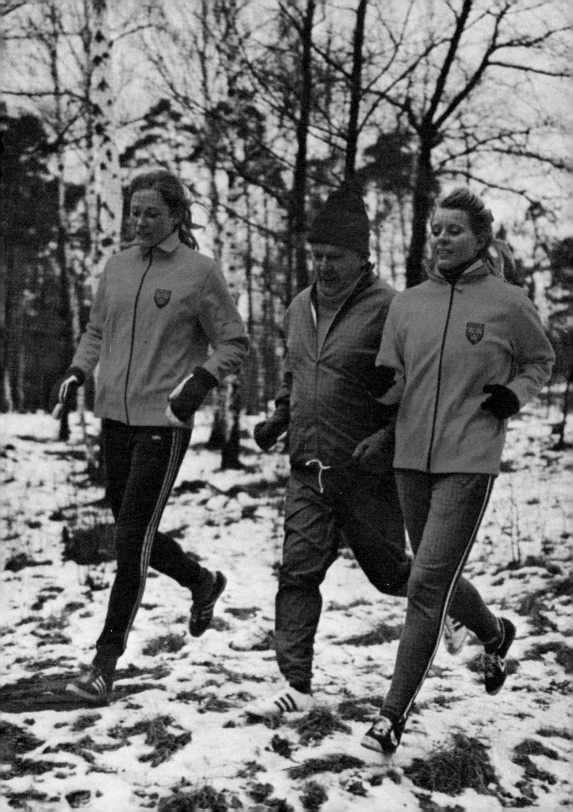

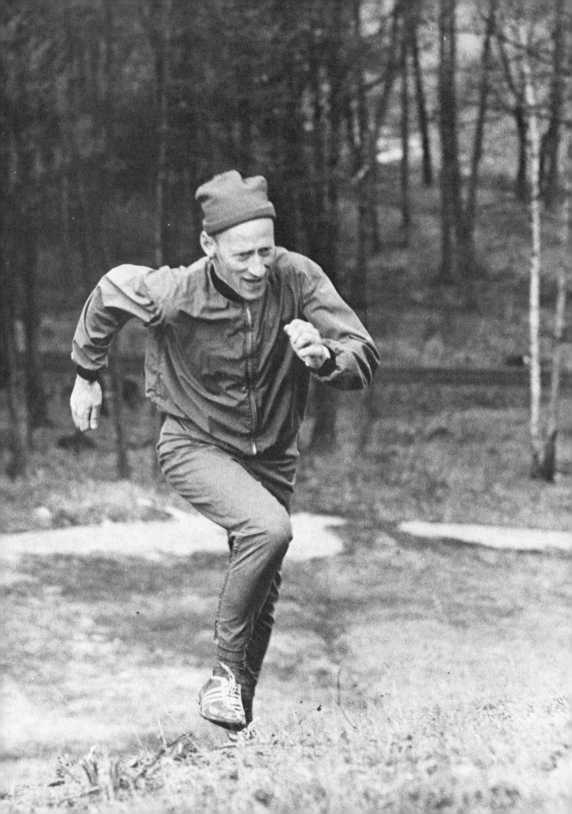

Foreword

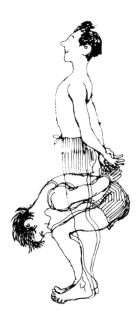

It is a great pleasure to publish this book *Health and Fitness* written by the eminent Swedish exercise physiologist, Dr. Per-Olof Åstrand. Dr. Åstrand originally wrote this book in Swedish for the Swedish people but what he had to say to Swedes applies equally to Americans, since the lack of fitness is an international problem.

Dr. Åstrand has spent a lifetime in the study of how we humans exercise. Besides being a scientist of worldwide repute, he is an excellent writer who can explain, clearly and with vitality, how our bodies respond to exercise.

The benefits of exercise are hard to comprehend without firsthand experience.

All the testimonials about how exercise can help a person feel and look better, cope with stress better, reduce mental and physical fatigue, and enjoy the social aspects of physical activity are meaningless until you participate and discover them for yourself. It is our sincere hope that some of this information will prompt you to include regular physical activity as a necessary but enjoyable part of your life. This book is one step in the direction toward becoming concerned about your life-style and stimulating you to do something about it. We hope that, after reading this book, you will understand how exercise can improve your fitness, and that a maintenance of an adequate fitness level is essential for positive health throughout life.

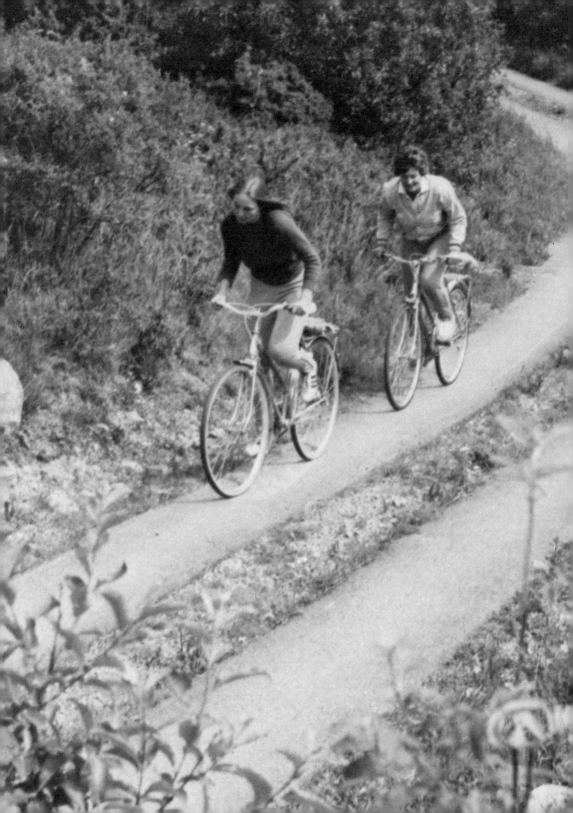

Introduction

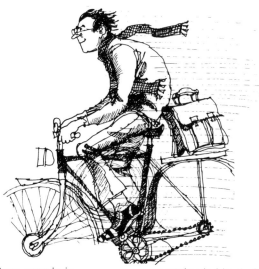

During the past century, people in industrialized countries have radically reshaped the environment in which they live. Technical devices of all kinds have assumed an increasing amount of the work formerly performed by muscle power. In most cases, changes were for the better. But they have also created major problems.

One of these problems is that the individual, originally designed for hard physical labor in the Stone Age, must adapt to a world dominated by technical innovations. Modern men and women must appreciate that regular physical activity is necessary if they are to function properly. Part of the ample spare time that we all enjoy — as compared to previous generations — must be utilized for active reaction.

Many dangers threaten if we do not follow this advice: a reduction in the capacity of certain vital body functions, obesity, malnutrition, an increased risk of contracting certain diseases, reduced resistance, and general fatigue. However, we are by nature rather lazy creatures, gamblers who take high risks in the hope that we are the exception to the rule, that everything will work itself out for us in the end.

This is why emphasizing the dangers of smoking, alcohol, narcotics, and general physical inactivity is seldom effective. People devote more attention to maintaining the good condition of their cars and their pets than to their own health. But it is of vital importance that we should be physically fit in order to manage our daily work and make our leisure time meaningful. Two or three half-hour periods of rational training every week are sufficient to build up and maintain good physical fitness.

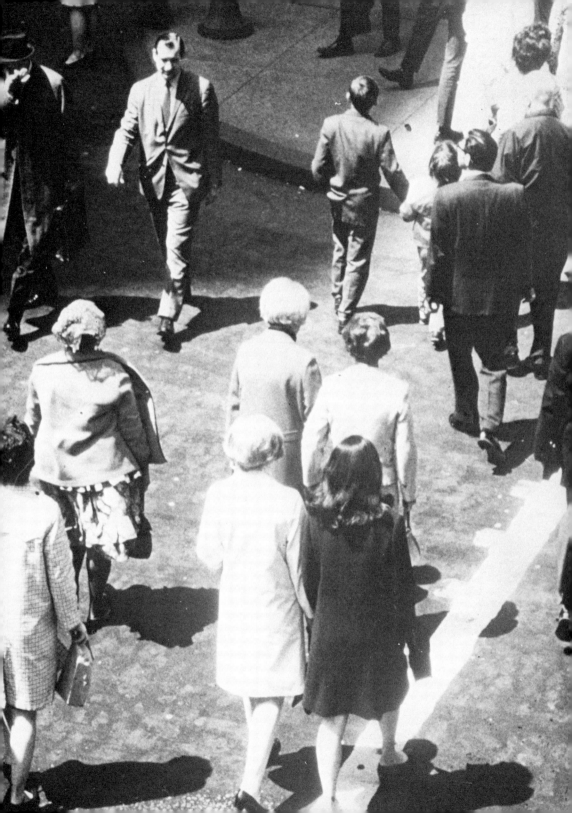

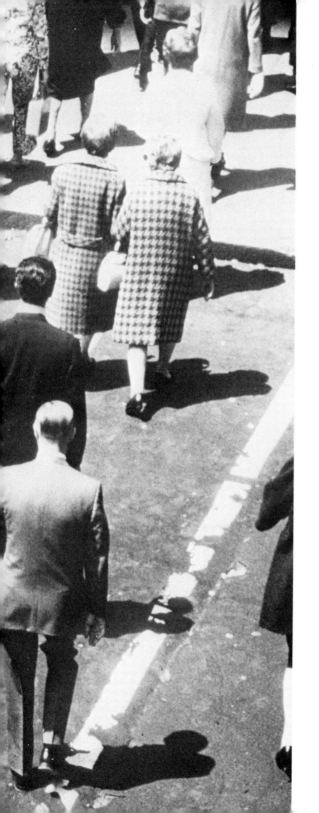

The American scene

Americans are unfit. Recent studies to determine the fitness of the average American showed that we are below the norms of the Scandinavian countries and that many Americans had fitness levels which could be classified as below those set by the American Heart Association. Unbelievable as it may seem, women are less fit than men, with teenagers and 20- to 29-year-old women rated the lowest.

Not only adults suffer the effects of indolence; most American children are also unfit. In a 10-year longitudinal study of school children, it was found that cardiovascular fitness declines steadily from the age of eight, stabilizing, at a very low level, only in late adolescence.

In the face of this evidence, it is not surprising that Americans are also fat. The average estimates are that over one-half of the adult American population is overweight. However, what is surprising is the finding that those who are fat eat the same number of calories as those of normal weight. Since our weight is a balance between the energy, in calories, that we eat and the energy that we expend in exercise, the problem of obesity must lie with our sedentary life-style.

Unfortunately in our society, we need only minimal amounts of physical activity to get us through the average working day. Even if we want to exercise, the temptations of inactivity are too great. Our automobiles tempt us away from walking, the elevators dissuade us from taking the stairs, and, most importantly, the television takes our interest from another activity that might use up a little energy.

The way in which we eat, exercise, smoke, drink, and drive — in short, the way in which we live — has a significant influence upon our risk of contracting many diseases. In a sense, many of the major health problems in America, such as coronary heart disease, automobile injuries, cancer of the lung, etc., can be considered diseases of choice. The responsibility for the prevention of these life-style health problems lies with ourselves. Unless we change, there is little hope that, despite the efforts of our health care system, we as a nation will improve our collective health.

People often ask, "Should I have a medical check-up before I start training?" The answer must be that people who are in doubt about the condition of their health should consult their physician. But as a general rule, moderate activity is less harmful to the health than inactivity. You could also put it this way: a medical examination is more urgent for those who plan to remain inactive than for those who intend to get into good physical shape!

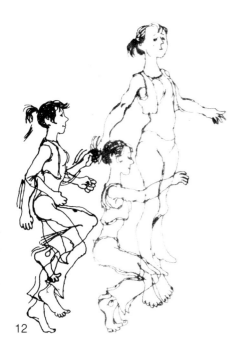

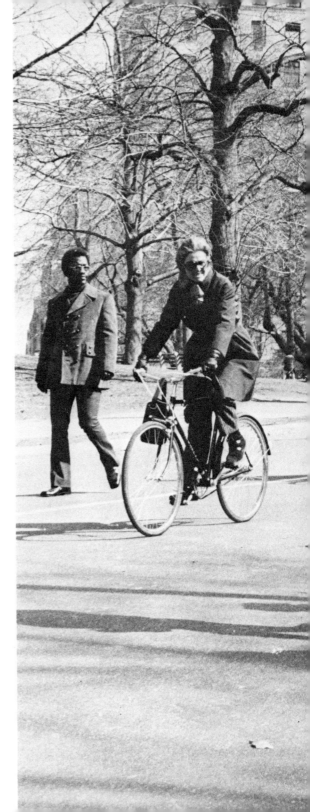

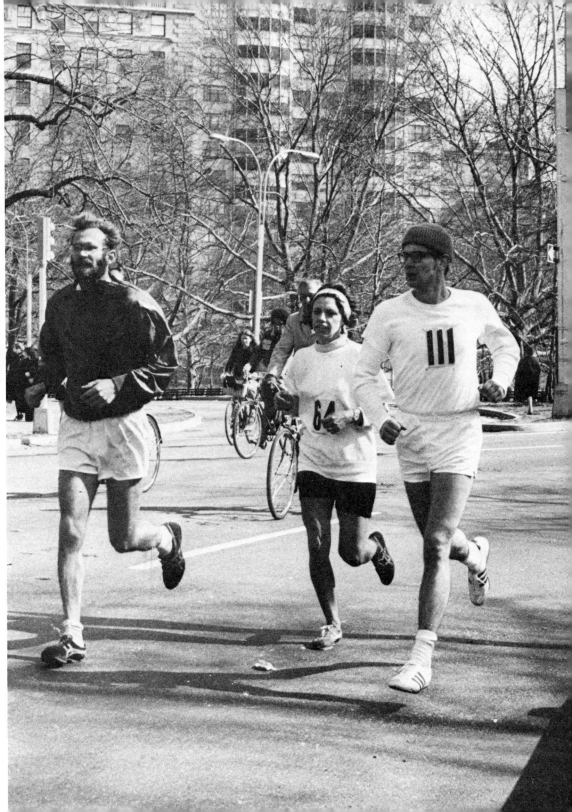

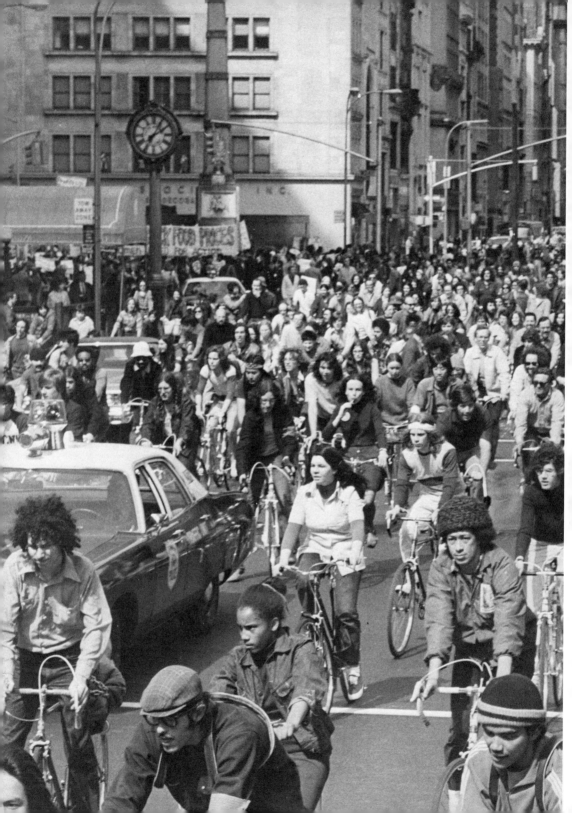

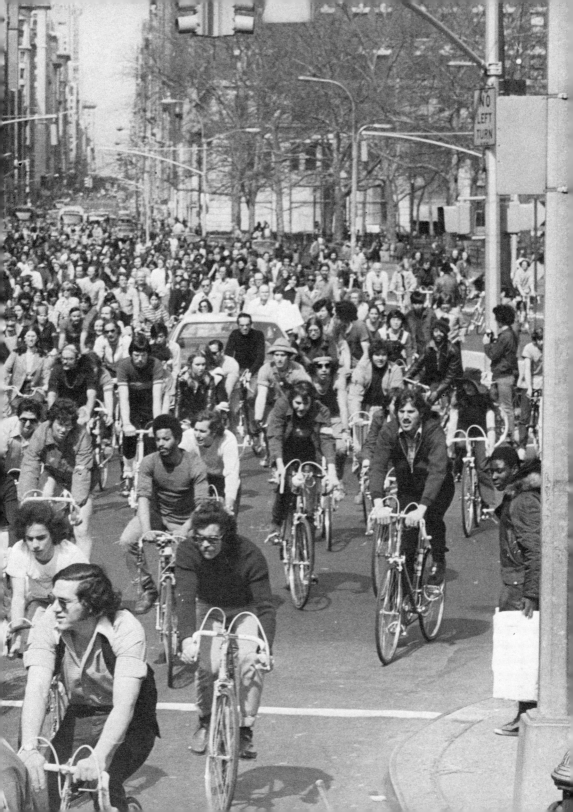

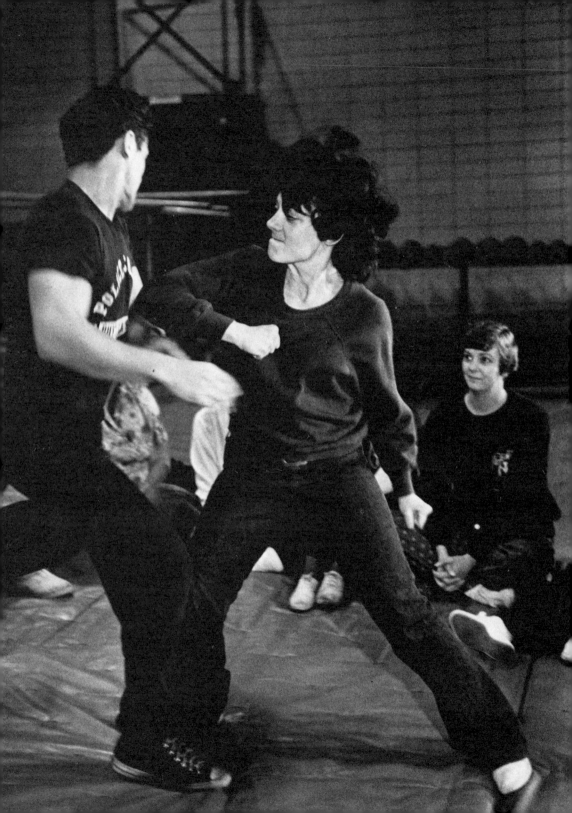

The human body – a working machine

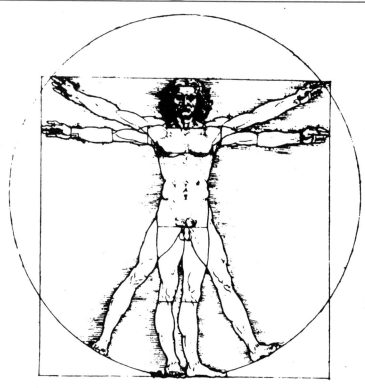

In most animals, the demand for good mobility dominates body construction. This also applies to human beings. The human body contains more than 600 muscles; overall, it is more than half muscle. Muscles make possible every overt motion. They also push food along the digestive tract, suck air into the lungs, tighten blood vessels to raise blood pressure when you need more pressure to meet an emergency. The heart itself is a muscular pump. Technological advances have changed our way of living and have made strenuous physical exertion largely unnecessary but the needs of the human body have not changed. Muscles are meant to be used.

Many of our important organs and functions are dimensioned and designed to give service to the muscles during work — organs such as the heart and respiratory system. With the body at rest, the heart pumps out about 5 liters of blood every minute and at the same time from 5 to 8 liters of air are inhaled by the lungs. Keep in mind, however, that the heart's construction permits it to pump from 15 to 20 liters (or more) of blood per minute and a person's pulmonary ventilation may exceed 100 liters per minute. The nervous system can also be said to be dominated by the body's demand for motion. To a large extent, the nerves receive and provide impulses that result in muscular movements: speech, gestures, physical work, running, etc., depending on the situation.

We're built for action

The human body is built for action, not for rest. This was a historic necessity; the struggle for survival demanded good physical condition. But optimal function can only be achieved by regularly exposing the heart, circulation, muscles, skeleton, and nervous system to some loading; that is to say, training. In the old days, the body got its exercise both in work and at leisure. In our modern society, however, machines have taken over an ever increasing share of the work elements which were formerly accomplished with muscular power alone. Our environment has come to be dominated by sitting, riding, and lying. Thus, the natural and vital stimulation that tissues and internal organs receive through physical work has largely disappeared.

That we are, to a great degree, what our muscles make us — weak or strong, vigorous or lethargic — is a growing conviction among medical men. Offering strong support for this conviction is the following observation by a former president of the American Medical Association: "It begins to appear that exercise is the master conditioner for the healthy and the major therapy for the ill." A recent survey of physicians showed that almost all now believe strongly that positive health benefits, both physical and mental, accompany physical fitness resulting from regular, moderate exercise.

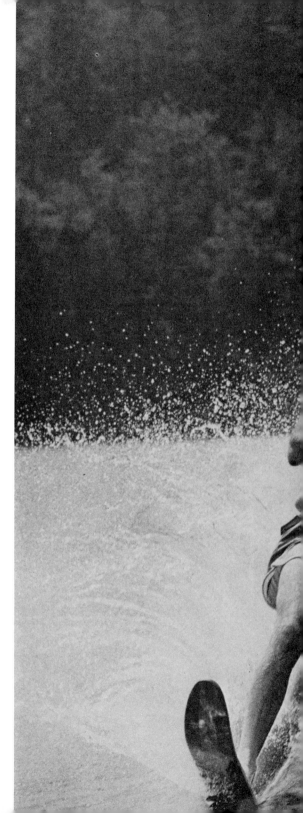

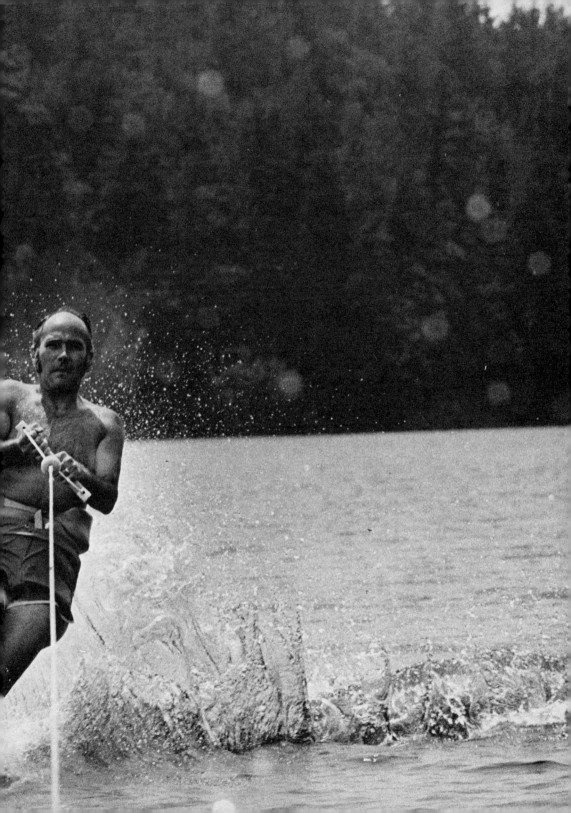

Prevent trouble before it could begin

Paul Dudley White, the noted heart specialist, once said that "prevention of disease has attracted much less attention than its diagnosis and treatment. It obviously deserves the first priority, but it is less dramatic than surgical procedures, is rarely asked for by the not-yet-educated public, and the doctors are overworked simply taking care of sick people."[1]

In many countries, cardiovascular diseases often account for more than 50% of all deaths. Naturally this fact motivates the intensive research presently being carried out to discover the genesis and treatment of such diseases. They certainly cause personal suffering and their social and economic consequences are enormous. In many countries, medical care is actually one of the largest industries, with a direct budget that has increased enormously during the past decades. In America, cardiovascular disease costs more than 22.7 billion dollars annually. In Sweden, with a population of 8 million, the health budget covered by direct tax revenue is now close to four billion dollars.

However, more money spent does not inevitably equal better health. Longevity, measured as the average remaining lifetime, increased markedly in America in each decade from 1900 to 1960 but appears to have reached a plateau in the early sixties. Since that time, there has been virtually no increase for males and only a slight increase for females.

Admittedly, life expectancy is in no way an accurate reflection of the state of health of a country. Life expectancy is determined from the death rate, whereas we measure our health, not when we die but while we live. The health of a country can only truly be measured by the quality of the life led by its citizens.

It is unrealistic to permit the cost of medical care to increase at the same rate as during recent decades. It would soon consume the total gross national income. Instead, much more effort and time should be devoted to preventive health programs. This booklet presents a summary of the physiological and medical information which analyzes the connection between health and fitness. This

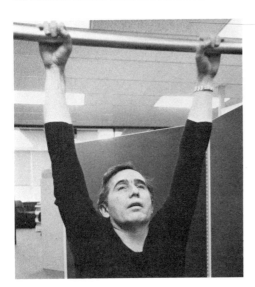

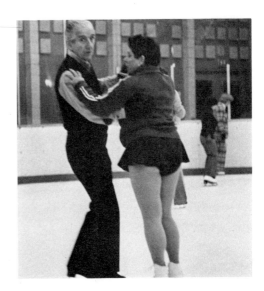

type of message has proved to be quite successful — at least in Sweden!

Actually, the increase in life expectancy over the past 70 years is largely due to a reduction in deaths of infants. In fact, the life expectancy of a 40-year-old man over the past half decade has increased by merely one year! Many diseases, particularly infectious diseases, have effectively been conquered, but diseases of a degenerative nature, particularly cardiovascular disease, have increased extensively. One cannot avoid the thought that our modern way of life could be one important factor and that the main determinants of longevity are now more cultural than medical.

In recent years, interest has been focused on the possible role of physical inactivity in the genesis of these diseases. The pioneer in studies of the "epidemiology" of cardiovascular diseases, J.N. Morris, has emphasized that "habitual physical activity is a general factor of cardiovascular health in middle age, and that coronary heart disease is in some respects a deprivation syndrome, a deficiency disease."[2]

Why exercise?

Athletes need to train to improve performance, but why should the rest of us keep in shape? As you will see from the following pages, the human body has been built for movement and that movement is a prerequisite for good overall bodily function. Regular exercise can be compared to the lubrication of a car. The regular lubrication keeps auto parts moving freely and exercise aids the overall performance of our body. In certain situations, good physical condition can even save lives; for example, in emergency situations in the wilds or under stress. However, the aim of regular training and exercise is not to produce great maximum strength but to achieve the essential by-products which training provides. Just what these by-products are is explained in the following pages.

[1] Paul Dudley White, *My Life and Medicine* (Boston: Gambit Inc., 1971).
[2] J.N. Morris and M.D. Crawford, "Coronary Heart Disease and Physical Activity of Work: Evidence of a National Necropsy Survey," *Brit. Med. J.*, 2: 1485, 1958.

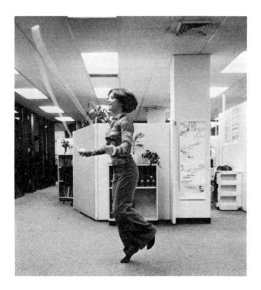

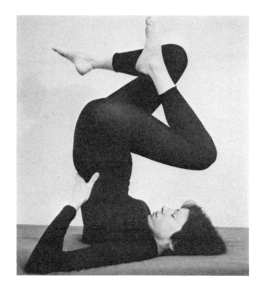

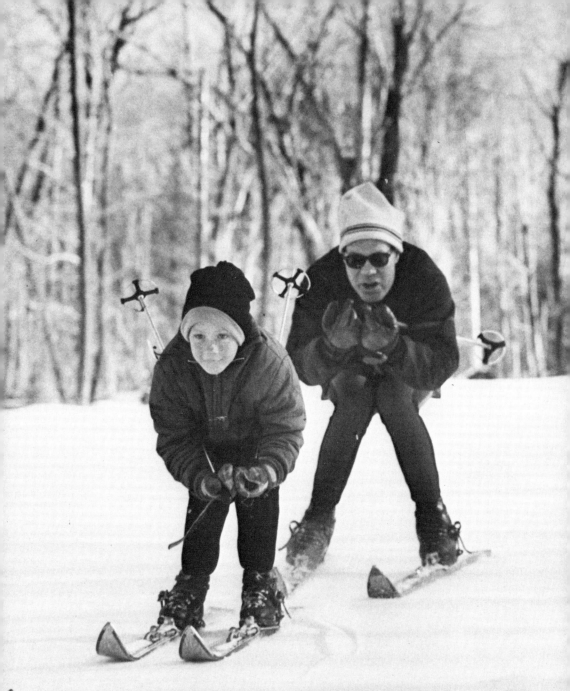

"... if the heart rate rises to 200 minus your age in years, a good training effect is being achieved."

The need for physical activity

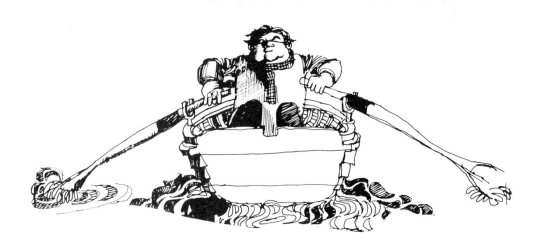

The saying goes: "You can get used to anything." This is, indeed, a fortunate attribute for human beings. You can get used to heat, cold, high altitudes, heavy work. But you can get used to inactivity, as well. The latter represents the reverse side of the coin. The problem is that we are scarcely aware of what happens to our bodies when we are too inactive. Today, various sophisticated methods of study have disclosed major, and sometimes dramatic, changes in our bodies as a result of inactivity.

Your body adapts to inactivity

If we are habitually inactive — if we succumb to the philosophy of easy living — we must then pay the price in decreased body efficiency. The most extreme form of inactivity is continuous confinement to bed. In a particular study, volunteers who submitted to bed recumbency for weeks at a time reacted with skeletal decalcification, reduced blood volume, reduced muscular

23

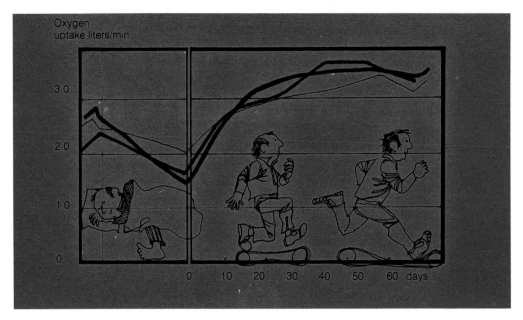

Fig. 1. The effect on maximal oxygen uptake of continuous bed rest for three weeks followed by rather intensive training. The three subjects were habitually inactive before the experiments. Note the 100% difference in the power of the "combustion engine" when comparing the data after training with that after bed rest. These changes reflect the variation in the heart's ability to pump blood.

mass, and impaired ability to take up and transport oxygen due to reduced stroke volume and cardiac output (Figure 1). They also displayed a marked increase in heart rate, at rest and also when working. This latter situation is one of the most easily detected changes as a result of inactivity.

Let's look a little further into exactly what happens when a person begins to feel the effects of prolonged inactivity. A job that would normally have been accommodated by a heart rate of 120 beats/min may, after several weeks of continuous bed rest, require 170 beats/min. The reason for this is that the body requires a given level of cardiac output, the product of stroke volume and heart rate. Reduced heart muscle strength and less efficient regulation of blood circulation will reduce the stroke volume and therefore contribute to this rise in the heart rate. After a

long period of inactivity, you may feel dizzy and may even faint when standing up. Your heart must compensate for this impaired stroke volume by beating more rapidly. In such a situation, the heart muscle requires more energy and a greater blood supply with this increased heart rate.

This rapid decline in physical condition creates very awkward medical problems, particularly when quick rehabilitation is desired. Anyone who has had an arm or leg in a plaster cast for some time has surely observed how rapidly muscular mass, power, and mobility are reduced. In many cases, rational physical exercise during convalescence can rapidly restore the patient's ability to work. Geriatric care would also be more effective if older people could be activated and trained to work in some way. This problem of inactivity is a severely neglected social and economic issue.

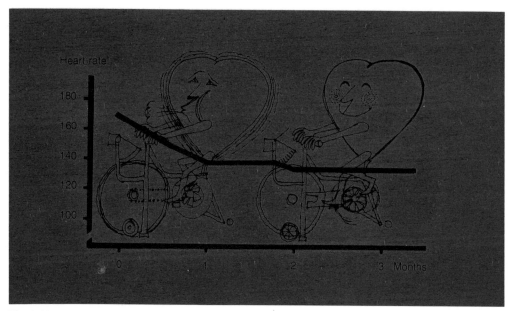

Fig. 2. Heart rate after approximately five minutes work on a bicycle ergometer (load 150 watts) in conjunction with three months of training. Note that heart rate gradually declines thanks to training of the heart.

Increased exercise means decreased heart rate

Any muscular activity requiring increased oxygen uptake will also lead to a strengthening of the heart and circulation; that is, to an improved physical condition. The effects of increased activity are just the opposite of inactivity. Muscular mass, blood volume, the power of heart muscle, and even the number of blood vessels all increase with exercise. If a relatively inactive person has a heart rate at rest of 70 beats/min, exercise can reduce this rate to 60 or less. A job that previously required a 170 beat/min heart rate can be managed with a 150, 140, or less rate, depending on the intensity of the training (see Figure 2). With a lower heart rate, the work being done by the heart is more efficient and less demanding. Unfortunately, active training is the only realistic "medicine" that can induce this beneficial effect physiologically.

Studies have been made which involved the monitoring of people's heart rates continuously for a 24-hour period. Such recordings have shown that even moderate training (as suggested in this book) can save some 10,000 to 20,000 heart beats per day. The exercise itself costs only some 2,000 extra heart beats per day. The actual medical consequences of this are difficult to evaluate but the figures are of great interest as an illustration of how heart work can be modified.

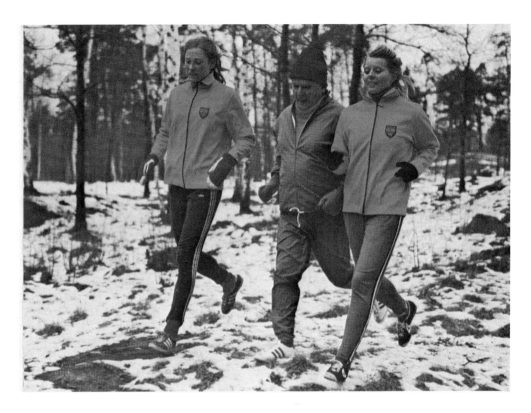

Cardiovascular diseases

Cardiovascular diseases are the cause of more than every second death in most industrialized countries. Naturally, intensive research is being done to investigate the cause of these disorders and how they can be counteracted. They certainly cause personal suffering and their social and economic consequences are enormous.

Arteriosclerosis is a chronic disease characterized by a thickening and hardening of the walls of the arteries. The first traces of arteriosclerotic changes in the blood vessels can be found in many teenagers. If those changes have not reached an advanced stage, they are reversible. When well established, however, the condition is much more serious. It should be pointed out that

several factors, such as heredity, diet, and way of life, seem to be of importance in the development of cardiovascular diseases. Individuals showing high blood pressure or obesity or a high concentration of cholesterol and triglycerides in the blood or a combination of these run a higher risk of death from cardiovascular diseases than those non-obese people with normal blood pressure and a low cholesterol and triglyceride level.

In studies published so far, it has been shown that inactive individuals run a risk of death from cardiovascular disease which is two to three times greater than that run by the active. The probability of surviving the first heart attack is statistically two to three times greater for those who have previously been physically active than for those who have been inactive. These are, of course, statistical correlations and do not prove that the degree of physical activity has actually been the sole and decisive factor. The studies were carried out on selected groups of individuals, and it is possible that certain factors that determined choice of profession or degree of activity during leisure time may also have independently given rise to some sort of prevention against cardiovascular diseases.

There are, however, physiological explanations as to how physical activity could be beneficial. Investigations on animals and observations of men have revealed that physical training can open up more blood vessels in the heart muscle; that is, additional branches may develop in the coronary arteries. Similarly, additional branch vessels may develop in peripheral arteries. A narrowing, or occlusion, of a vessel due to arteriosclerosis will not have the same consequences if there are other vessels that can take over the transport of blood with its necessary oxygen and nutrients to the tissue nearby the damaged vessel.

Regular physical activity will also favorably influence the level of triglycerides and possibly of cholesterol in the blood, particularly in patients with elevated blood lipid levels.

Research in this area is very complicated and it may take a hundred years or more of intensive study to demonstrate with certainty that there is or is not a connection between cardiovascular diseases and habitual inactivity. The question is then whether we should wait so long for final proof or whether we should consider the preliminary results. In my opinion, there is much indirect evidence that regular physical activity, or training, has a beneficial effect on the functioning of the heart and that the opportunity must be seized now. We should actively work to affect health in a positive way through a systematic improvement in physical fitness.

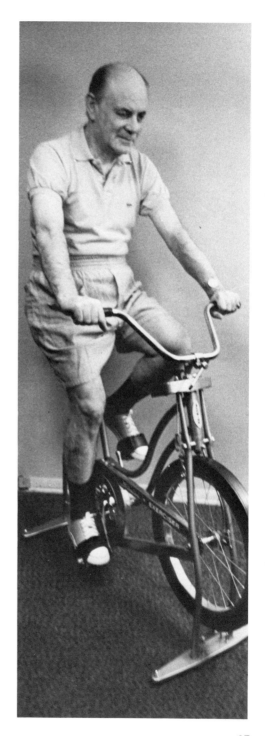

Back troubles

Diseases in the spinal column rank very high on the list of common diseases. They are responsible for many days of sick leave and thus give rise to economic problems and cause much related suffering. When a load is lifted or carried, a reflex mechanism calls the trunk muscles into action to fix the rib cage and to compress the abdominal contents. The intra-cavitary pressures are thereby increased and aid the support of the spine. Scientific observations emphasize the important role that the trunk muscles have in supporting the spine. While flabby abdominal muscles may leave the spine exposed to injurious stress, well-developed abdominal muscles, on the other hand, are an important protective device that can prevent damage to the spinal column and help avoid possible resultant backache.

To be sure, the trunk muscles probably have no influence on the inevitable changes in the spinal column that come with age, but if they are well developed and trained, these muscles can, to a great extent, prevent the symptoms caused by the occurrence of a weak back. Walking or running upstairs or uphill will train the leg and trunk muscles. Simple but, if possible, daily exercises will also strengthen these muscles. As back troubles are so common, it is important that a person keep his or her trunk muscles fit. It is also important that everyone knows how to lift and carry loads in a way that reduces the load on the spinal column.

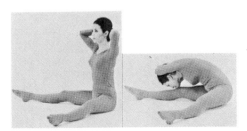

Chronic fatigue

Ranking today as one of the most frequently voiced of all complaints, chronic tiredness can stem from illness. But in many people, investigators report, it is the result of gradual deterioration of the body for lack of enough vigorous physical activity.

Continual inactivity produces muscular atrophy and the individual soon becomes under-muscled for his or her weight. The result: that person lacks the strength and endurance to do his or her daily work easily and efficiently.

One important end result of the increased muscular strength and general endurance provided by exercise is an increase in the body's capacity for carrying on normal daily activities, a pushing back of fatigue limits. Valid research indicates that a fit person uses less energy for any given movement or effort than a flabby or weak person.

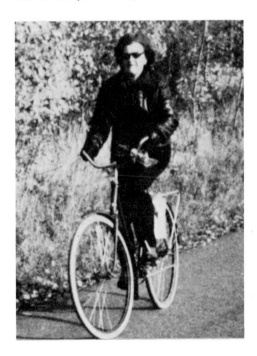

Aging

There is strong authoritative support for the concept that regular exercise can help prevent some degenerative diseases and slow down the physical deterioration that accompanies aging. The evidence is conclusive: individuals who consistently engage in proper physical activity have better job performance records and fewer degenerative diseases. By delaying the aging process, proper exercise also prolongs your active years.

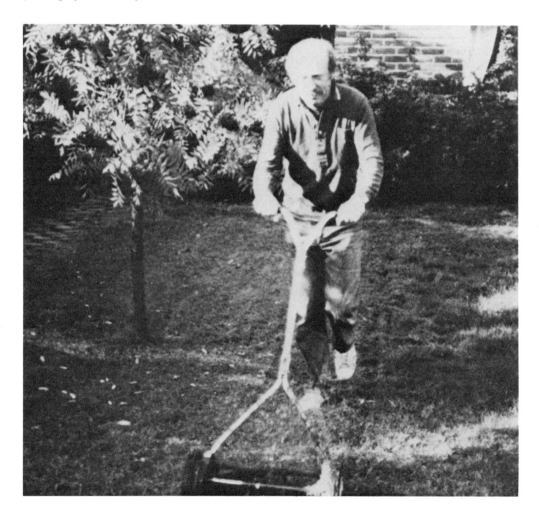

Obesity

A common misconception is that exercise does not aid in weight control. This is not the case. Research has shown that fat piles up in most people by only a few Calories* a day; that an excess of only 100 Calories a day can produce a 10-pound gain in a year's time; and that obese people almost invariably tend to be much less active than those of normal weight; and that individual weight is a factor in energy expenditure. If you are overweight, you will burn up more calories in performing exercise than a person of normal weight.

Inactivity is the most important factor explaining the frequency of "creeping" overweight in modern society. And the consensus now among medical authorities is that the most effective way to take off weight and keep it off is through a program which combines proper exercise and reasonable diet.

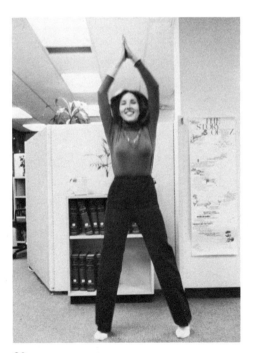

In summary

To summarize, certain tissues such as muscles, bone, and blood, and also a number of bodily functions, can adapt to inactivity — and to stress. Inactivity impairs the capacity for physical work, while a well-adjusted load improves it. Exercise can provide the following benefits:
- ♥ increased strength, endurance, and coordination
- ♥ increased joint flexibility
- ♥ reduction of minor aches, pains, stiffness, and soreness
- ♥ correction of remediable postural defects
- ♥ improvement in general appearance
- ♥ increased efficiency with reduced expenditure of energy in performing both physical and mental tasks
- ♥ improved ability to relax and to voluntarily reduce tension
- ♥ reduction of chronic fatigue

We are constructed for activity; we once had to run in order to survive and if we are to maintain ourselves in a state of optimum function, we must, from time to time, be physically active; we still have to run for our lives!

*The unit is kilocalorie (kcal); 1 kcal = 4.2 kilojoule (kj)

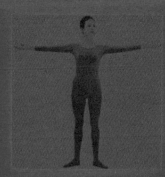

 # Fit tips

For your daily routine, add a little
fitness perspective . . .

Start each day with a stretch,
bringing your muscles into activity

Walk every chance you get — walk to
the next bus stop, walk the dog, walk
to the store

Eat and enjoy yourself but remember
to maintain your level of activity

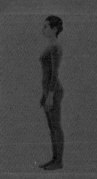
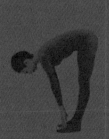

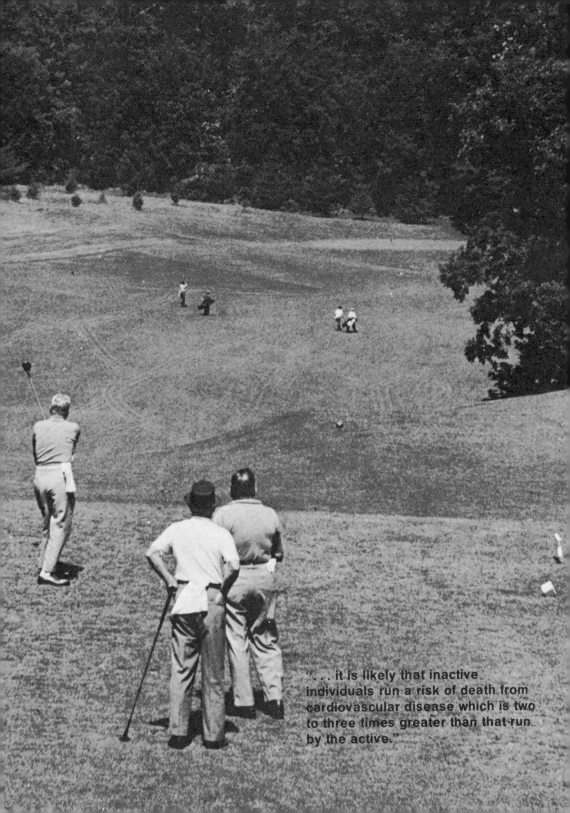

" . . . it is likely that inactive individuals run a risk of death from cardiovascular disease which is two to three times greater than that run by the active."

Energy yields and aerobic fitness

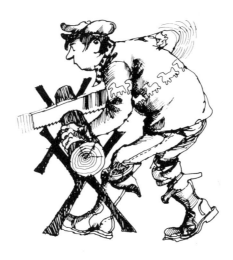

Every cell in the body is essentially like a combustion engine. The fuel that powers it is glycogen (a kind of carbohydrate) and fatty acids. The cell, like an engine, also needs oxygen to yield energy, and it produces carbon dioxide and water as "waste products."

When we breathe, we take air into our lungs. Breathing conducts air (containing about 21% oxygen) down to the alveoli (air cells) in the lungs. The hemoglobin in the red corpuscles of the blood then takes charge of the transportation of oxygen from the lungs to the cells throughout the body. In the cells of the various organs, the oxygen is exchanged for carbon dioxide, which is then carried back to the lungs by the blood stream and is then exhaled. For every liter of oxygen consumed by the body, a certain amount of energy — approximately five Calories or 20 kilojoules — is liberated.

In the initial phase of an activity or during some less strenuous exercise, the muscles can make use of an *anerobic* ("without oxygen") engine. The energy yield takes place in the absence of oxygen as the energy-rich substances (the fuel), including glycogen, are split up into less energy-rich substances, thereby releasing energy for muscle work. However, the ability of the body to work in this manner is very limited. This anerobic motor dominates in intensive muscular work for a minute or two, but the longer the duration of the work and the more intensive is the nature of the work, the more important it is for the combustion engine to attain a higher power output. This higher output can only be attained through *aerobic* fitness.

When the body is taking in oxygen to produce energy, it is utilizing aerobic power. Intensive exercise or extended activity requires such aerobic power and this involves a more efficient use of oxygen. Oxygen uptake can be measured when the body is either at rest or at work. If a subject performs a maximum effort for five minutes on a bicycle ergometer or treadmill and the oxygen uptake is monitored, a measure of the maximum power of the "combustion engine" is derived. Since oxygen is transported by the blood, the figure for oxygen uptake also gives an evaluation of the load on the heart and circulatory system. The greater the maximal oxygen uptake (technically called the *maximum aerobic power*), the greater the heart's ability to pump.

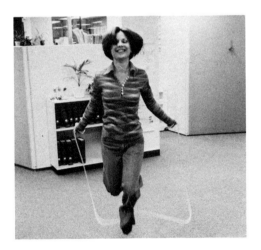

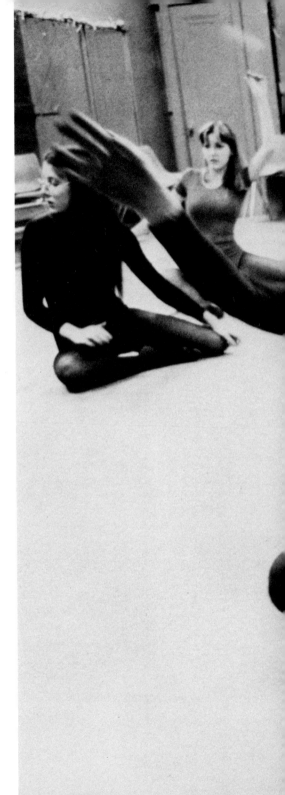

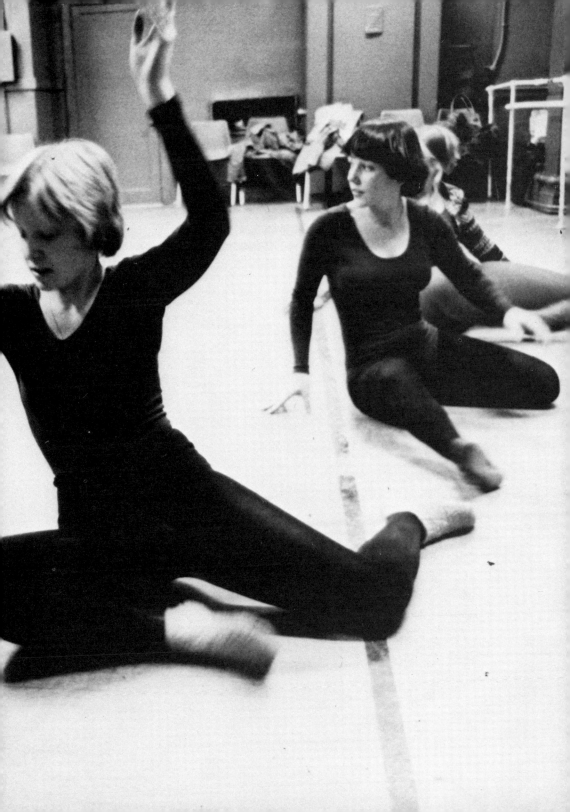

Increasing your maximum oxygen uptake

It is desirable for a person to work to increase his or her maximum aerobic power. By doing so, a person can strengthen the muscles involved in respiration, increasing the ease with which air flows in and out of the lungs; such conditioning will also improve overall circulation and increase the pumping efficiency of the heart. Exercise can increase a person's maximum oxygen uptake by 10 to 20% or more. It should be noted, of course, that natural endowments do play a great role in providing a human engine with high power and that a completely untrained person may have a maximum oxygen uptake which is greater than the mean value indicated in figure 3. A well-trained person may have a lower maximum oxygen uptake than the average, accordingly, with a low level of performance.

The effects of age

Figure 3 shows how maximum oxygen uptake (and indirectly the cardiac function) changes with age in moderately well-trained persons from 4 to 65 years. The highest value is achieved in the twenties and the curve then falls, so that a 60-year-old has about 70% of the value of a 25-year-old. Studies have proved that, with regular training, a person can counteract (if not completely prevent!) the decline in maximum motor power which usually accompanies increasing age beyond 20. We would put it this way: if two 50-year-olds are identical in endowment but one is trained and the other untrained, then the trained person would have an oxygen uptake ability (and maximum motor power) on the same level as the untrained person had around the age of 35 or 40. In other words, moderate training can lead to a 10- to 15-year biological rejuvenation in this respect.

There may be many reasons for the decline in maximum oxygen uptake with advancing age. Gas exchange in the lungs becomes less efficient, maximum breathing capacity decreases, and the gas exchange between the lungs and the blood becomes less efficient. Since the elasticity of blood vessels declines, demands on the heart's pumping ability increase at the same time as the blood supply to the heart's own muscle drop off. Maximum heart rate drops from about 200/min in youth to about 160/min around the age of 70. The muscle mass and maximum muscle power also decline.

Part of this decline is the inevitable result of aging, but it is also probably a consequence of our changed way of life. Sports and relatively strenuous outdoor life have been replaced by more sedentary activities. The body does not take long to adapt itself to reduced demands which impair work ability. It may also be a question of a chronic malnutrition, but regular exercise and improved diet can counteract this decline.

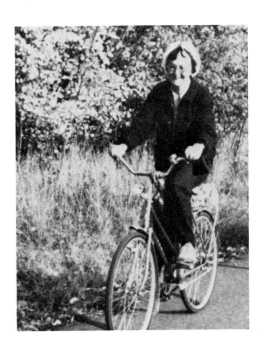

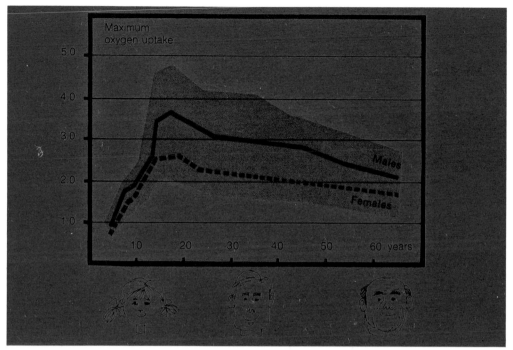

Fig. 3. Maximum oxygen uptake changes in this way for healthy, moderately well-trained persons from 4-65 years.

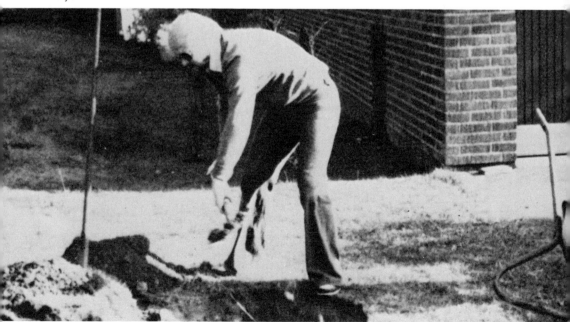

Differences in sex

Before the age of 12, the values for boys and girls are very similar. But after puberty, the maximum aerobic power of boys is greater than that of girls. On the average, women's values are 25 to 30% lower than men's. However, the differences among individuals is often greater than the differences between the averages for the sexes. Top-class women athletes produce maximum motor power greater than most men; a 25-year-old woman has, on the average, values greater than a 65-year-old man. On the other hand, a 65-year-old man may, owing to personal characteristics, have higher values than a 25-year-old woman. Professions traditionally considered physically unsuitable for women may be equally unsuitable for older men.

Psychological factors

Sometimes we may be in the mood for physical exercise and sometimes not. In certain situations we feel that we could move mountains but at other times nothing seems to work.

Certain areas of the brain hold a key position in the question of coordinating muscles. Activity can be influenced by, among other things, a person's mood. As a rule, muscle cells cannot be brought to maximum contraction with the aid of willpower alone. But, in certain situations, such as through the influence of hypnosis, the promise of reward in conjunction with strong encouragement, or in situations of danger, strength may increase beyond normal limits (some sort of emergency reaction). Thus, the ability to perform may vary from day to day without any change in the training status or without the influence of illness. Moreover, not everyone is equally interested in heavy physical labor. Some people actually like to torture themselves, bringing their bodies to a point of extreme stress, while others are lazy and give up as soon as they start to feel physical resistance.

Work tactics are also of great importance. A person with severely impaired respiratory, cardiac, or circulatory function can manage rather heavy work if he or she takes frequent micro-pauses; that is to say, 10- to 30-second rest pauses interspersed with equally long periods of work.

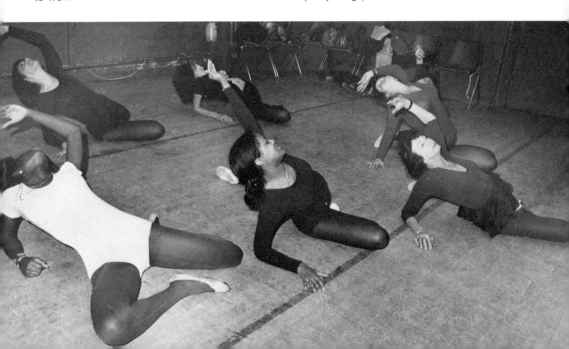

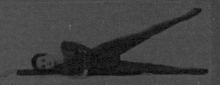

 # Fit tips

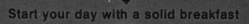

For a better exercise session:

♥

Start your day with a solid breakfast

♥

Try doing several short exercises
during the day if you don't have time
for one longer one

♥

Exercise to music, for better rhythm
and more enjoyment

♥

Add to your exercise quota by
learning new sports and trying other
activities that you might enjoy

♥

Relax your muscles after every
exercise session

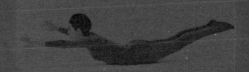

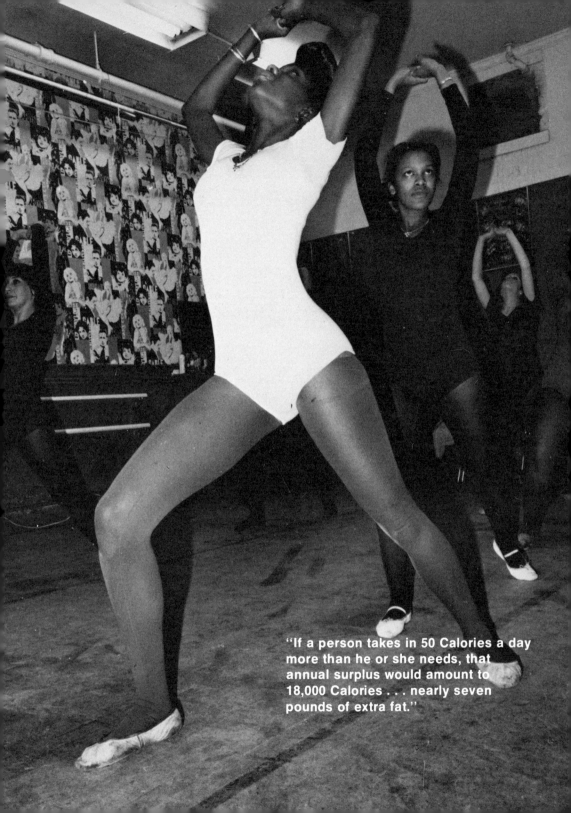

"If a person takes in 50 Calories a day more than he or she needs, that annual surplus would amount to 18,000 Calories . . . nearly seven pounds of extra fat."

Weigh what you weighed in your twenties

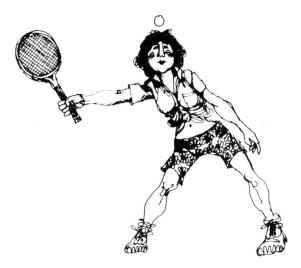

People tend to put on weight after they reach the age of 25, an aesthetic problem which can also be a health liability. There are no simple height-weight tables that can indicate with certainty if a person's weight is normal for a particular age or if he or she is overweight or underweight. A heavy person may weigh a great deal without excess fat, while a light person may be obese. A good rule of thumb is that a person's weight should not increase after he or she reaches the twenties. Since muscular tissue declines in most of us, a loss of a few pounds after age 20 is actually good proof that there is no increase in fatty tissue.

Limit your intake to lose weight

Sensational new findings regarding dieting turn up at regular intervals in newspapers, magazines, and books. Sometimes the recommendation is to avoid fats; sometimes carbohydrates get the blame for overweight. The actual truth is rather simple: if the energy intake corresponds to the energy expenditure, body weight does not change except for small variations of up to a couple of pounds (1 kg) a day which may occur, mainly due to fluctuations in the body's water content. All excess energy is converted into

41

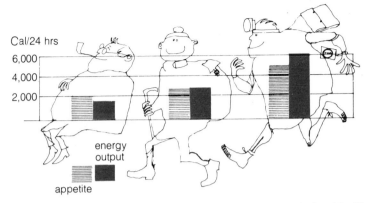

Cal/24 hrs
6,000
4,000
2,000

energy
output

appetite

Fig. 4. The diagram shows three persons with different levels of habitual physical activity. The man to the left moves very little and "burns" no more than 1,800 Cal/day but his appetite "demands" some 2,000 Cal. He has to accept being hungry if his weight is not to increase.

The man in the middle is more active and has a balance between his appetite and energy output.

The cross-country runner to the right can symbolize a very active day. He "burns" more Calories that he is interested in eating up.

fat. It matters little if the energy is in the form of fat, carbohydrates, protein, or alcohol (Figure 4).

How many Calories should you consume?

Obesity is only occasionally due to pathological or organic disturbances. Both fat children and fat adults are actually just less physically active than people with normal body weight. Two pounds (1 kg) of fat correspond to about 6,000 Calories. A person with a sedentary occupation and little body movement during leisure needs from 1,500 to 2,500 Calories a day, depending upon body size. Athletes in hard training and people engaged in heavy manual labor consume up to 5,000 Calories a day. Thus, energy output per day varies between the amounts of energy represented by 11 ounces up to about two pounds of fatty tissue. Energy requirements are usually met rather closely by the corresponding supply of energy in the form of food and beverages.

But with habitual inactivity, the appetite is often set for an energy supply greater than the need. We could put it this way: we can choose between being habitually inactive but often hungry or being fairly active and therefore able to eat most of what we like!

Extra weight goes on slowly

If a person takes in 50 Calories a day more than he or she needs, that annual surplus would amount to 18,000 Calories, corresponding to nearly seven pounds of extra fat. This could eventually lead to a 70-pound weight increase in ten years. If you should one day decide to eliminate a routine activity, such as a mile walk each day, but you maintain your same eating habits, you are likely to gain 100 pounds in ten years (Figure 5). It's not surprising that obesity's approach is stealthy as life becomes more sedate, thanks to the automobile, and as we assume more sedentary jobs with less time devoted to exercise. In this context, the period between 25 and 30 years of age is rather critical.

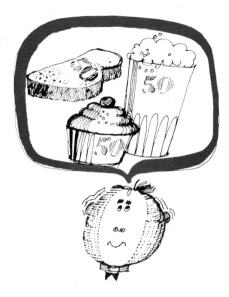

Fig. 5. 50 Cal extra/day leads to nearly 7 lb (3 kg) weight increase in a year. The form in which the extra Calories are ingested does not matter.

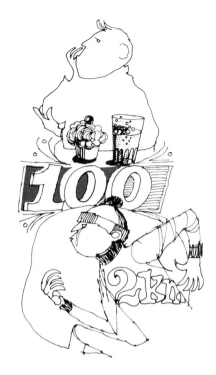

Fig. 6. A brisk walk, jogging or running ¾ mile corresponds to an energy cost of 100 Cal.

Adjusting your menu

The most gentle way to reduce weight involves allowing plenty of time for the measures you use to take effect. Menus should be critically examined for opportunities to substitute lower-calorie foods or to eliminate certain high-calorie items entirely. For example, about 100 Calories can be eliminated by excluding sugar or replacing it with an artificial sweetener; ordinary milk can be substituted with low-fat milk. Furthermore, you can use up additional energy by adding a 1.5-mile walk to your daily habits. The results of such measures would correspond to an approximate total of 200 Calories difference. If everything else remains the same, after a month, the body will be holding 6,000 Calories less than before, the equivalent of about two pounds of fat. Twenty-five pounds should have been eliminated in one year, if the schedule is maintained (Figure 6).

If rapid results are desired, increased exercise can be combined with a strict diet so that only 800 to 1,000 Calories a day are eaten. That would be a tough program, however, because there is no diet that is low in energy but which still leaves you satisfied. Weight loss is often striking the first few days, but this is mainly due to loss of body water and not to a loss of fat. It should be pointed out that fat cannot be massaged or kneaded away, nor can it be shifted from one place to another.

In summary, any person hoping to lose weight will find that increased physical activity and a change in diet from one rich in fat and sugar to one containing relatively more protein is the most dependable, acceptable way to achieve that end (Figure 7).

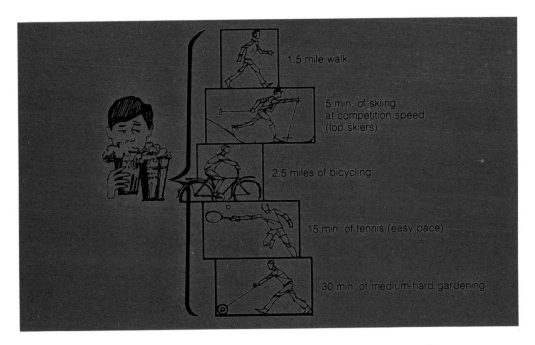

Fig. 7. It's easy to feed 100 Cal to the body but difficult to burn them, as the drawings illustrate.

A proper diet is important

Studies have shown that many individuals often live on a diet with fewer than 2,000 Calories a day. These people are often habitually physically inactive and they do not need more than 2,000 Calories to meet their meager energy needs. However, with a traditional diet, an intake of more than 2,000 Calories a day is necessary to satisfy the body's need for enough vitamins, minerals, and proteins. Although such people manage to maintain an acceptable weight limit, they may be depriving their bodies of necessary nutrients. In addition, if a person's diet, however many Calories are consumed, has a preponderance of foods with low content of vital substances (which is likely to be the case in a diet of mainly fats, sugar, sweets, snacks, cookies, and cakes), the risk of malnutrition and disease is strong.

Some 25% of the women in the world suffer from iron deficiency anemia. In some areas of the United States, it is also reported that up to 60% of the female teenage population have an intake of some vitamins below the recommended amount. Indeed, some of our "modern" diseases, including arteriosclerosis, may partly be consequences of chronic malnutrition. It is a mistake, for example, for people limiting their intake of energy to avoid carbohydrates completely (potatoes, bread, rice) because muscles and nerve cells need carbohydrates in their metabolism. This is particularly important for anyone who is also physically active.

The best way for people to guarantee an adequate diet is for them to combine high-energy consumption with increased physical activity. Thereby, they can eat more and automatically get more of the essential

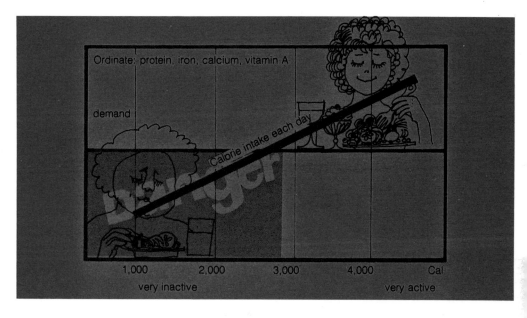

Fig. 8. The supply of most essential nutrients is roughly linearly related to the daily energy intake, but the demand of such nutrients remains constant. The risk for malnutrition is minimal among high energy consumers; i.e. the physically active person.

nutrients. Eating is one of the true pleasures in life; if you are physically active, you may eat more without becoming obese. So, in summary, those who are habitually inactive must watch their diet very carefully and select food items rich in essential nutrients (Figure 8).

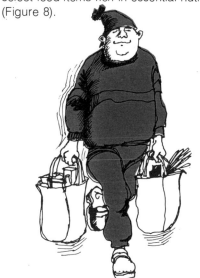

How does drinking liquids influence your weight?

Some people feel that they should drink as little as possible when exercising and when it is very hot because if "you drink just a little, you perspire less." However, studies have shown that sweat production is rather independent of the body's fluid balance. Moreover, sweating is the mechanism that prevents overheating of the body when it is warm or when heavy work is performed. Therefore, under such conditions, sweating is very desirable. If fluid is not replaced at the same rate it is lost, performance capacity and fitness decline and the feeling of exertion increases. Heart rate and body temperature rise abnormally. You should, therefore, drink deliberately, possibly even more than your thirst "orders" when you sweat. But you should not drink too much at a time nor drink very cold drinks.

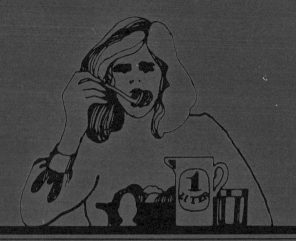

 # Facts on food

**Combine your cut-back in calories
with an increase in exercise to
achieve a maximum weight loss.
Following is a typical plan for a
200-Calorie diet difference:**

activity	Calorie difference
5 flights of stairs at the office, 3 flights at home, twice a day	35 expended
One 1-1/4 mile walk home from the bus	100 expended
Replacement of whole milk with low-fat milk (8 oz.)	40 less
Reducing the layer of butter or margarine on bread/sandwiches by half	25 less
	200 Calories eliminated from your daily count

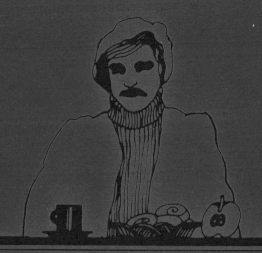

 # Facts on food

Your nutritional needs: Be sure to include each of the following in your diet.

meat — beef, veal, lamb, pork, variety meats, poultry. Fish and shellfish. Alternates: dry beans, dry peas, lentils.

vegetables — all fruits and vegetables as a source of vitamins A and C.

milk — all dairy products, including whole and skim milk, buttermilk, cheese, ice cream, yoghurt.

bread-cereal — whole grains, enriched or restored, including breads, cereals, cornmeal, crackers, grits, macaroni, noodles, rice, oats, bulgur.

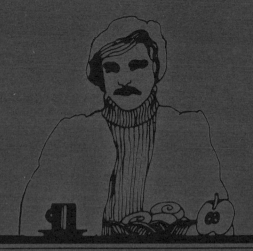

 # Facts on food

Try another plan to eliminate 200 Calories from your daily total:

activity	Calorie difference
1-1/4 mile walk	100 expended
Use of artificial sweetener instead of 4 cubes of sugar	50 less
1 less cookie a day	50 less
	200 Calories eliminated from your daily count

Here's another plan:

activity	Calorie difference
Replace a potato with an extra portion of vegetables at dinner	75 less
1/2 a dinner roll instead of the whole roll	75 less
Half a glass of beer instead of the whole glass	50 less
	200 Calories eliminated from your daily count

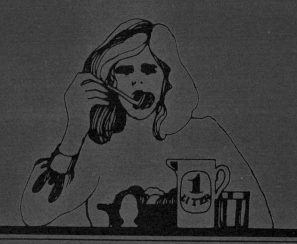

 # Facts on foods

Following are the energy contents for certain foods:

food item	energy content*
4 cubes of sugar	50
1 chocolate bar (plain)	200
1 slice of a fruit pie	550
1 cookie	50
1 hard roll	150
1 piece of iced layer cake	350
1 slice of white bread	70
10 peanuts	60
1 apple	90
1 chicken leg	90
1 3 in. hamburger on a bun	500
1 8 oz. glass of beer	110
1 8 oz. glass of ale	130
1 oz. of Scotch	80
1 Martini (average)	160

* 1 kcal = 4.2 kj

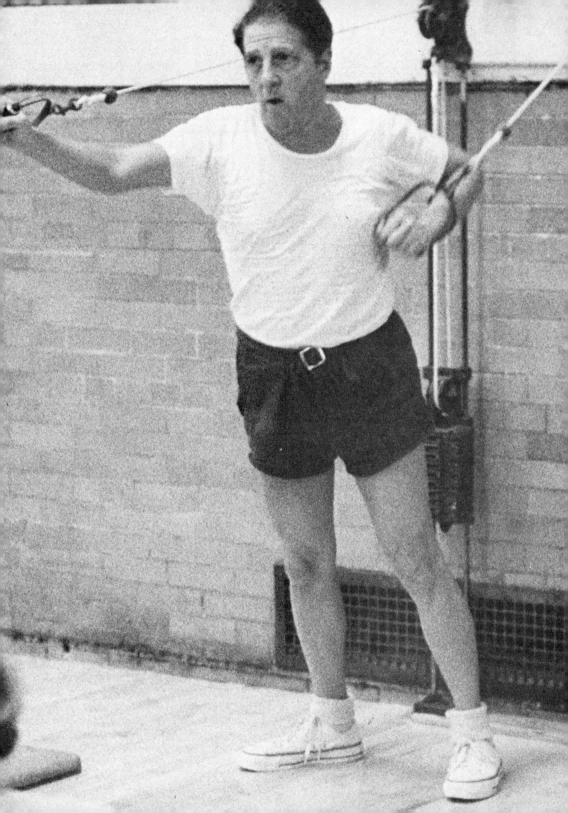

Getting into shape

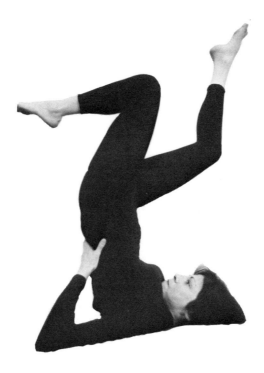

Physical fitness for everyday life

One important aim of regular physical training is to achieve a physical condition and fitness that is well above that required for routine jobs. This way your body is properly trained to serve you when you need additional fitness, such as times of stress of vigorous activity. If daily work forces a person's heart to pump ten liters of blood a minute, with a 120 beat/min heart rate, it is obviously advantageous for a person to be trained for 15 liters/min and a 150 beat/min heart rate or even more. In their spare time, people should give their bodies the stimulation in the form of exercise they need in order to function at their best and for their ultimate best health.

People who perform heavy manual labor daily usually are in better shape than average white collar workers. Manual laborers' jobs provides them with a certain amount of physical training and physically heavy work is absolutely no liability for healthy people. In view of this, a quick walk now and again may be sufficient for a teacher or office worker to move toward better fitness but a person who does heavy work should exercise even harder a few sessions a week.

Recreation as physical activity

By active recreation we mean a kind of hobby in which some form of muscular work is a big part. Examples of passive recreation are watching television, attending concerts or the opera, playing cards or chess, and collecting stamps. Both active and passive recreation are necessary for your well-being and both should be something to look forward to with joy and expectation.

Passive recreation should, however, also be supplemented by active recreation. Such a combination is birdwatching. You go out into the country with binoculars and a field guide to locate birds. The bird moves and you have to follow it to identify the species and to study details. Vigorous walking is often combined with restful watching and waiting periods.

If you are inclined to spend your evenings watching television, then combine this passive recreation with active recreation during the day. Examples of active recreation are gardening, hunting, fishing, and swimming. Unfortunately, many of these activities may be very much dependent upon the season. Therefore, some purposeful training in some form should be undertaken that will carry through the year. In selecting your activity, however, be sure that it is an enjoyable one for you. You shouldn't, for example, rush through the woods on your training round, trying so hard to beat your record that you are blind to all the surprises nature has to offer in those woods.

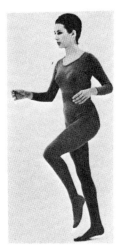

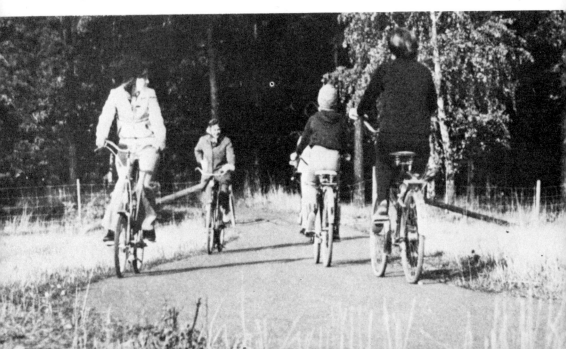

Starting a program

Walking at an easy pace improves physical condition somewhat, therefore people completely out of shape should begin at a gentle pace. Conditioning is more efficient, however, if the pace is increased as fitness increases. One effective training method is to have large muscle groups working hard — but not at maximum — for a few minutes. One should then rest or "take it easy" for a few minutes, work harder again, etc., three to five times. A quick walk, jogging, running, skiing, cycling, swimming, rowing, skipping rope, and jumping in place are good physical activities.

When a certain level of fitness has been achieved, a person should try to retain it. Training then feels gradually easier. Less training is required to retain good physical condition than is needed to acquire it. That's why regular training is so important. If you begin your "shake-up" by training every day or every other day for a few weeks, you can achieve good results that can be preserved without much effort.

A prescription for physical activity

Daily — at least 60 minutes of physical activity, not necessarily vigorous, nor all at the same time.

Weekly — at least two or three periods of 30-minute sustained activity (brisk walking, jogging, cycling, swimming, cross-country skiing, etc.).

Remember. . .

1 Be active: *move, move, move. . .*

Don't avoid a chance to walk rather than ride. Try whenever possible to be active. In doing so, you will be balancing the amount of energy you take in by eating with the energy you spend up by being active. The effects of physical activity are cumulative: short periods of activity add up to a lot during the course of a day. If your daily schedule does not allow you an extended single period of activity, you may still obtain the desired amount each day by combining briefer sessions.

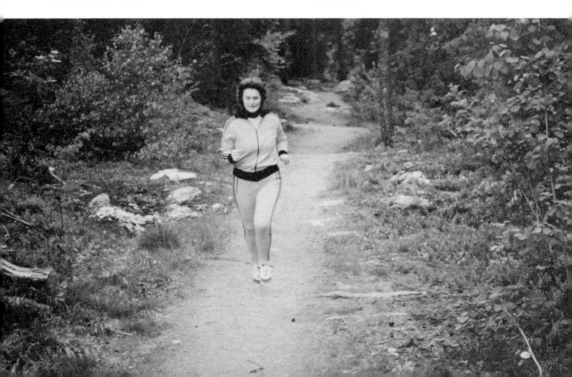

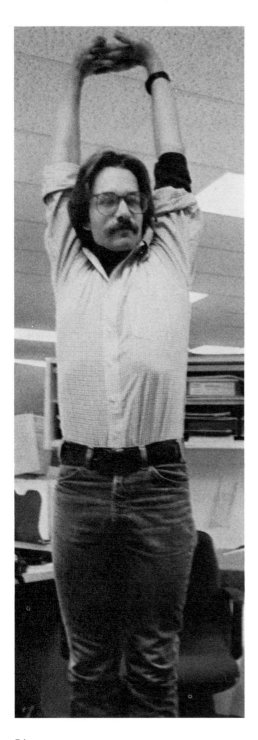

2 Stretch: *Give yourself a break, for your muscles' sake. . .*

Ever notice how a dog always stretches its body when it arises from a nap? After you have been sitting for an extended time, take a break and give your muscles a good stretch. Tighten the muscles in your arms and legs. Relax. Take a deep breath. Relax. You will be giving your muscles some needed use and you'll be ready to start concentrating again.

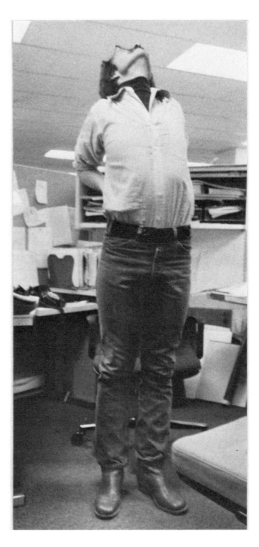

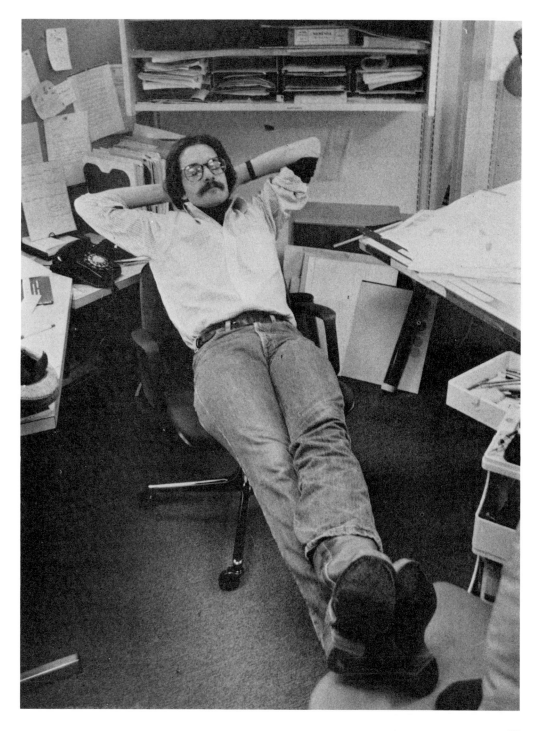

3 *Exercise:* *use your muscles...*

Keep your muscles in shape by doing a variety of exercises that require you to bend, twist, and swing your arms and legs. All this activity will help your muscles become more flexible and increase in strength. Your goal: to develop your coordination, expand the ability of your muscles, and improve the function of the joints.

Health and Fitness includes many suggested exercises that will increase your muscle flexibility. See pages 65-78.

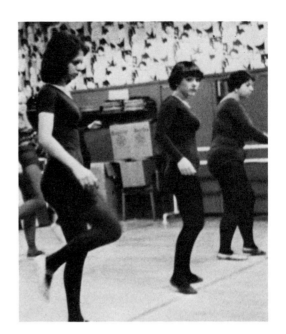

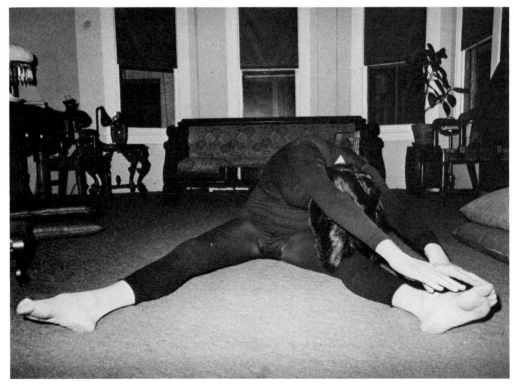

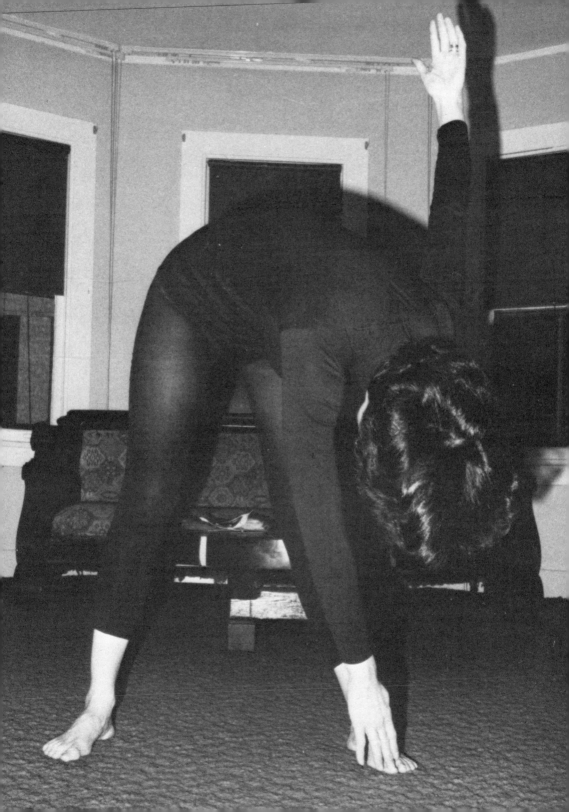

4 Work out: *short vigorous exercise sessions*

Your body also needs regular periods of brief but vigorous physical activity. Try to include such sessions (15 to 30 minutes) three or four times a week. This sustained vigorous activity will strengthen your heart and lungs.

Prescription for minimum aerobic fitness

Frequency — 3 times per week

Intensity — hard enough to make you perspire, breathe deeply, and increase your heart rate (see chart next page)

Time — 15 minutes of vigorous activity (using heart rate chart) preceded by adequate warm-up and followed by cool-down phase prior to shower

Type — endurance type activities which are rewarding, pleasant and preferably fun. i.e.: cross-country skiing, bicycling, snowshoeing, swimming, jogging, etc.

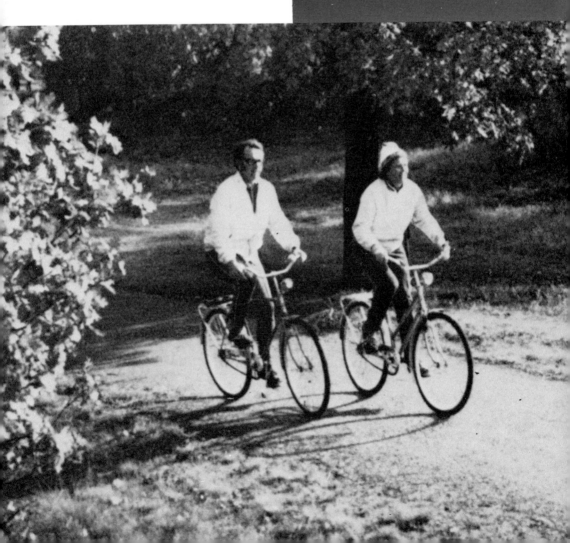

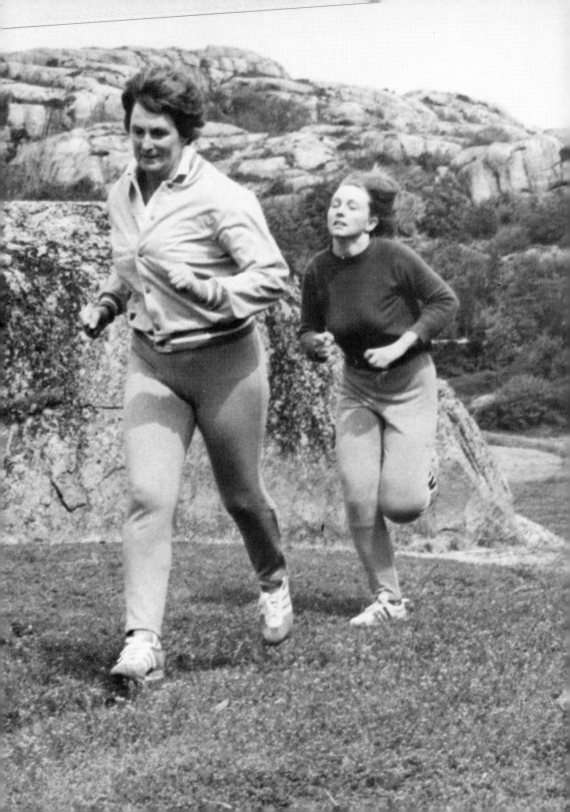

5 *The sporting life:* *make it a part of your life...*

Develop some interests in sports that involve active participation. Your body will enjoy the activity and your mind will appreciate the relaxation. Depending upon your age and circumstances, try jogging, swimming, skiing, walking — whatever you find pleasurable and whatever is suitable or practical for you.

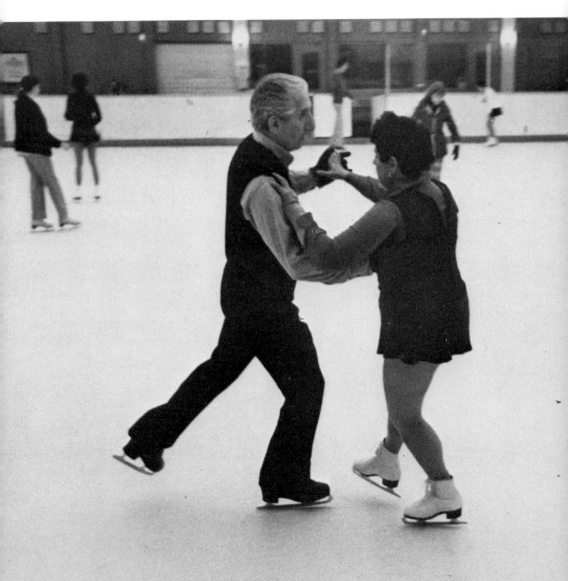

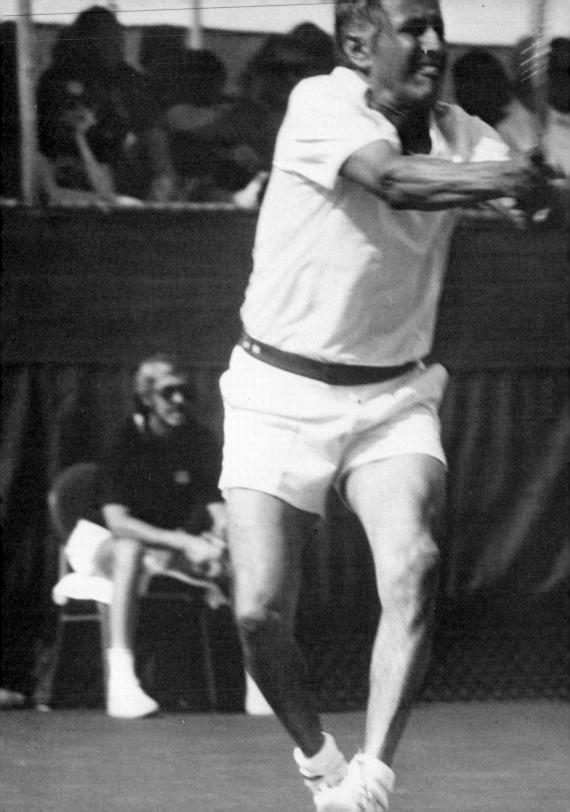

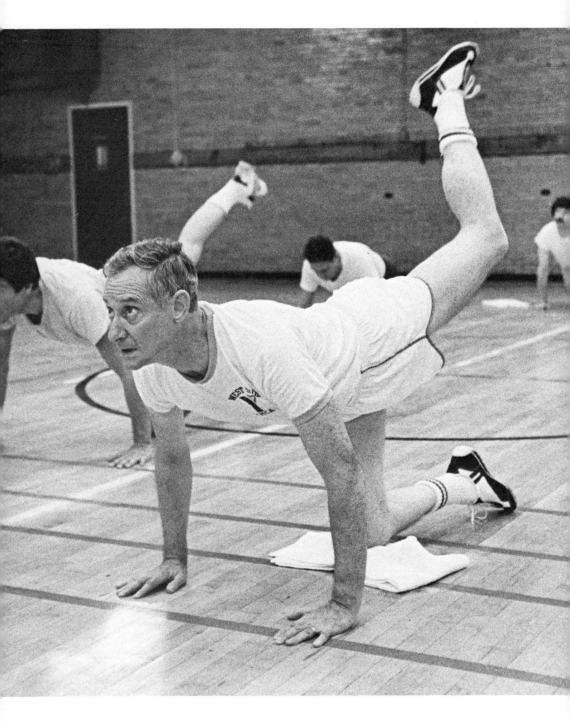

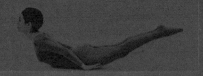

Fit tips

For some quick relaxation:

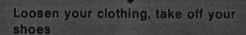

Loosen your clothing, take off your shoes

Stretch, lift your arms and try to touch the ceiling with your fingertips

Walk or lightly jog in place for a few minutes

Shake your shoulders and bend from your waist, first in front and then to each side

Bend your knees and touch the floor

Take a deep breath, relax

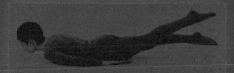

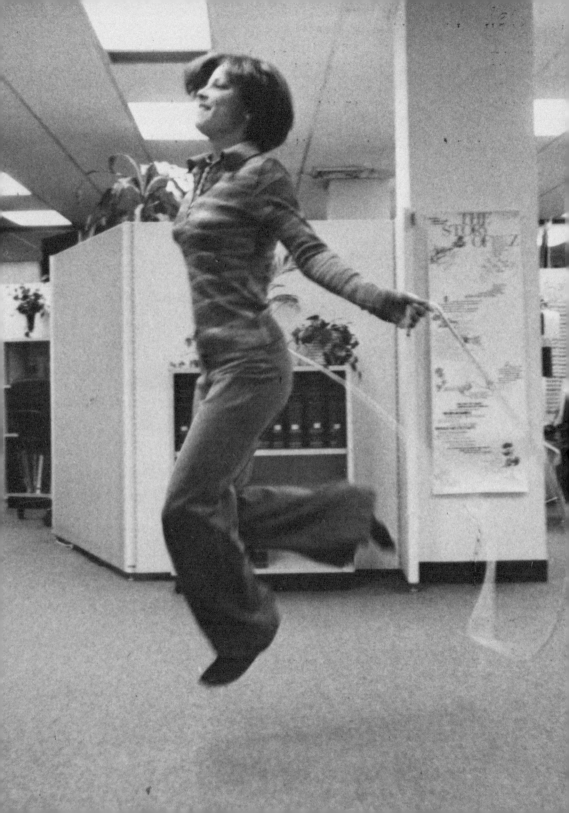

A training program for home use

Total time: 8 to 15 minutes.

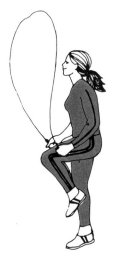

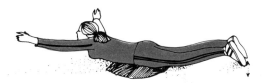

3. Lie on your stomach, preferably with a cushion under your pelvis. Lift your legs and upper trunk so that your body rests on the cushion. Keep your arms extended at your sides or stretched outward. Repeat the exercise up to 16 times.

1. Skip or run in place for one minute. Rest for half a minute. Then begin a new period of work for one minute.

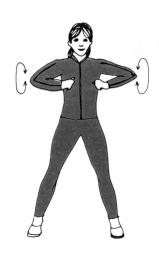

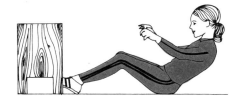

2. Sit on the floor with your knees bent and your feet supported. Lie down and sit up again. Repeat this exercise up to 16 times.

4. Stand with your feet apart. Do about 24 shoulder rolls. Change the direction of rotation every revolution or every fourth revolution.

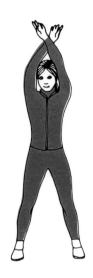

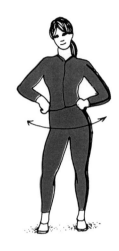

5.   Stand with your feet apart. Do about 24 arm swings across the front of your body as in exercise 4.

7.   Stand with your feet apart and your hands on your hips. Slowly rotate your hips.

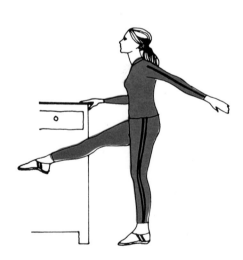

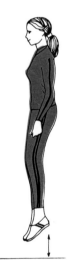

6.   Stand on one leg, supporting yourself with one hand on a table or other stationary object. Do about 24 leg and arm swings, changing sides every fourth swing. Try to raise up on your toes in the extreme positions.

8.   Skip easily in place or jog for a half a minute.

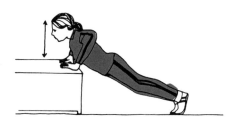

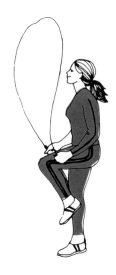

9. Lie on the floor. Extend your arms with your hands against the floor (strong and healthy persons) or against a sofa or chair (less fit persons). Do one to 15 push-ups keeping your body straight.

10. Skip or run in place or take the step test for one to five minutes.

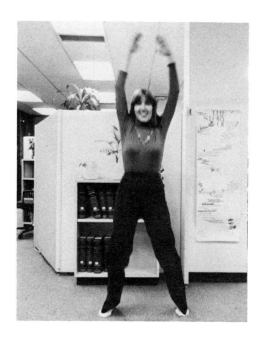

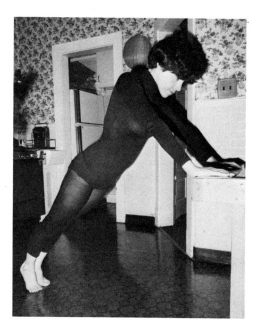

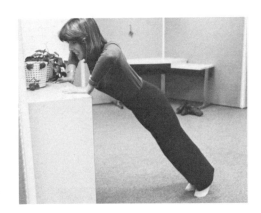

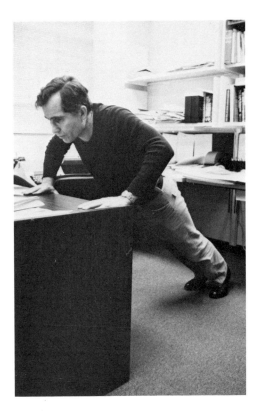

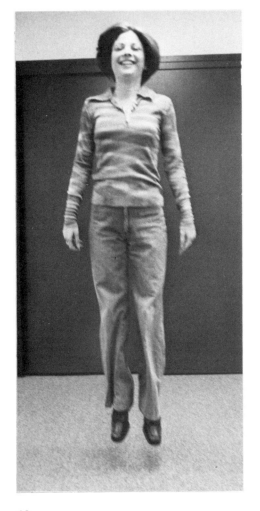

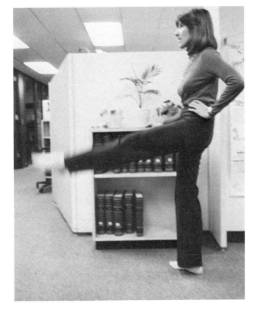

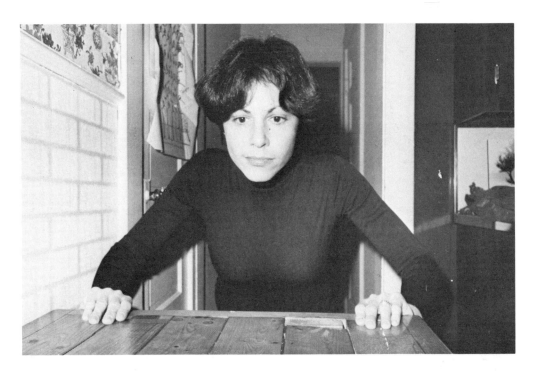

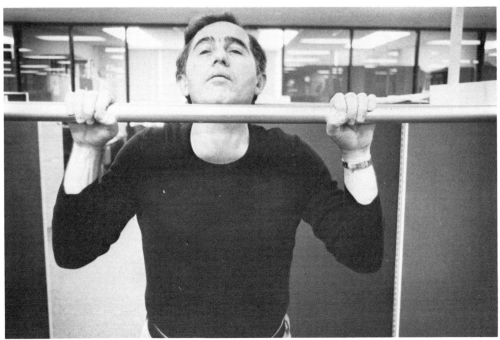

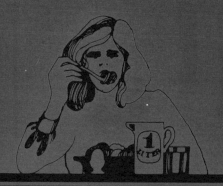

 # Facts on food

How much energy do you need to maintain weight?

weight (pounds)	minimally active (Calories)	moderately active (Calories)	highly active (Calories)
100	1500	2000	2500
120	1800	2400	3000
140	2100	2800	3500
160	2400	3200	4000
180	2700	3600	4500
200	3000	4000	5000

Following are examples of energy consumption:

activity	Calories expended
1/2 mile walk	40
1/2 mile jogging or running	80
5 flights of stairs	10
1/2 hour bicycle ride	200*
20 minutes of steady swimming	170*

*More or less, depending upon speed and, in bicycling, road surface and wind.

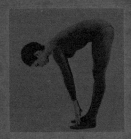

 # Fit tips

For a better daily diet:

Start your day with a good breakfast

Get your protein from yoghurt, cheese, meat, fish

Get your vitamins from fresh fruit and vegetables

Get your iron from dried beans, raisins, liver

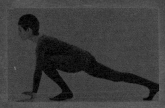

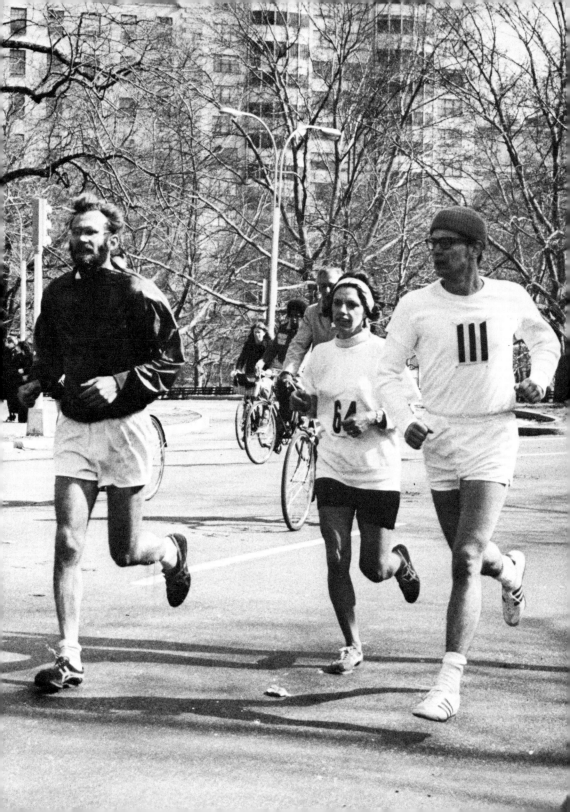

A training program for those in good physical condition

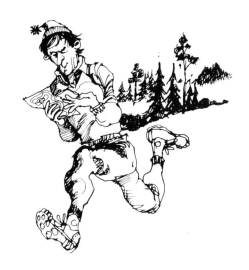

1. Five-minute warm-up. Alternate jogging and walking.

2. Five-minute spurt training. Run 20 to 30 strides at top speed about five times, preferably uphill.

3. Recovery between spurts.

4. 15 to 20 minutes of interval training. Run at about 80% of your top speed for two to four-minute periods. Rest or job between these periods.

It is convenient to arrange dressing rooms, simple playgrounds (for children's games, volleyball, table tennis, basketball, etc.) adjacent to the training tracks.

Personally, I like to change to suitable clothing at home and to drive out to the track. As a warm-up, I walk alternating with jogging for about five minutes. That takes me to a steep hill, which I climb with 20 to 25 steps at top speed, thereby loading the legs and buttocks muscles. I walk down, pause briefly, and begin a new rush up again, repeating this about five times.

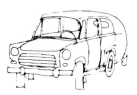 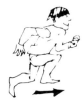

This phase takes about five minutes and is not as exhausting as it sounds since each work period is brief. Training of the cardiovascular function then follows with repeated three- or four-minute periods of running with a two to three-minute rest or easy walk in between. As I have already mentioned, maximum speed is not used; about 80% of capacity is the desired level. My training round comprises four "conditions sections." Some 30 to 35 minutes later, I'm back at the car and I drive home to enjoy a shower.

One suggestion: don't run downhill! The risk of injury is very great and the conditioning effect is rather modest.

". . . individuals who consistently engage in proper physical activity have better job performance records and fewer degenerative diseases."

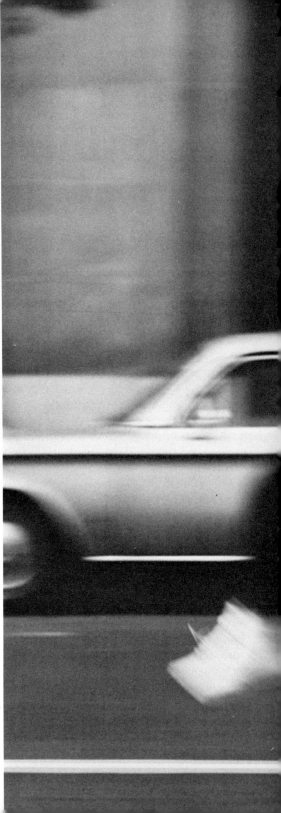

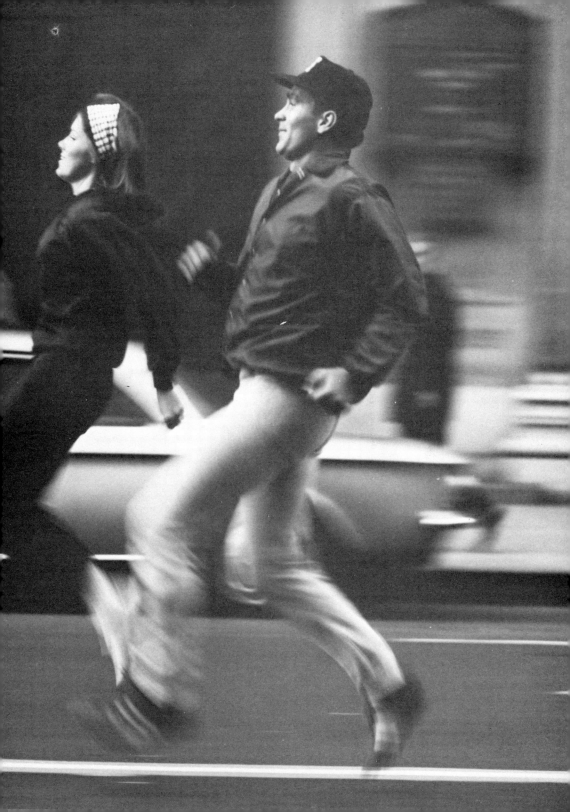

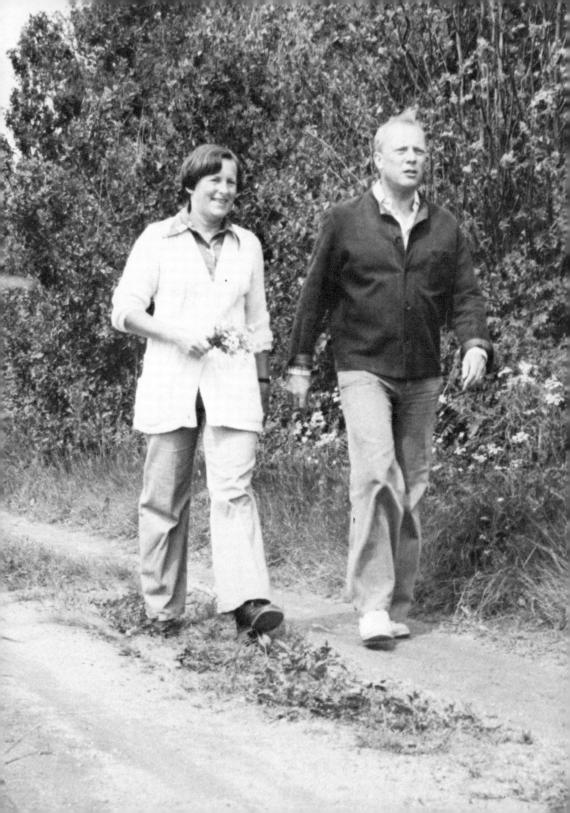

A training program for inactive or elderly persons

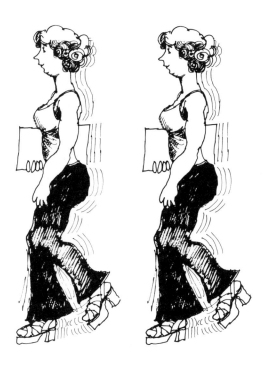

Where there is impairment or illness, any and all exercise should be medically prescribed and regulated. Today, physicians are using exercise as an aid in combating many chronic problems, including arthritis, asthma, diabetes, and emphysema. As mentioned previously, common types of low back pain have been traced to weakened back muscles, and exercise has been used both to produce relief and to help prevent recurrences. If you have a handicap, your doctor may find that some or many of the exercises given in this manual — perhaps with modifications — could be of value to you.

The following is a basic training program for those who cannot participate in more extensive physical activity. The basic pace is ordinary walking speed. Begin leisurely and gradually increase the pace, but not so fast that you become out of breath.

1. Five-minute warm-up. Walking.
2. Five-minute spurt training. Take 20 to 30 strides at a rapid pace, preferably uphill.
3. Recovery between spurts.
4. 15 to 20-minute interval training. Brisk walk for two- to four-minute periods. Rest or walk slowly between periods.

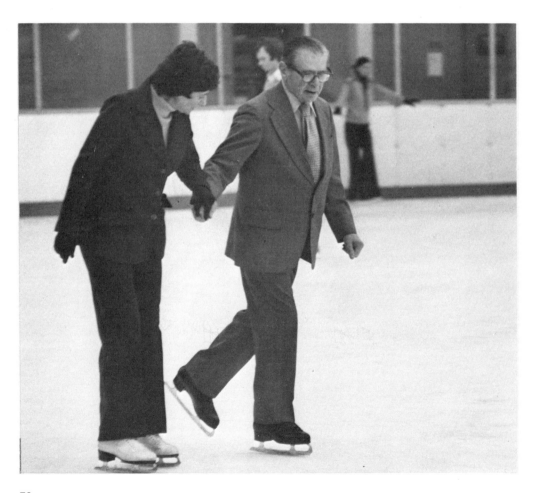

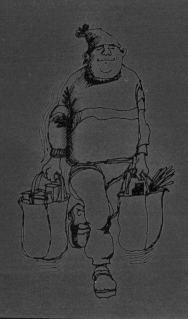

 # Facts about heart disease

Cardiovascular diseases cost
Americans $22.7 billion annually.

Approximately 29 million Americans
have some form of cardiovascular
disease.

Deaths from cardiovascular disease
comprise 52% of all deaths in the
United States.

About 350,000 persons die each year
of a heart attack before ever
reaching a hospital.

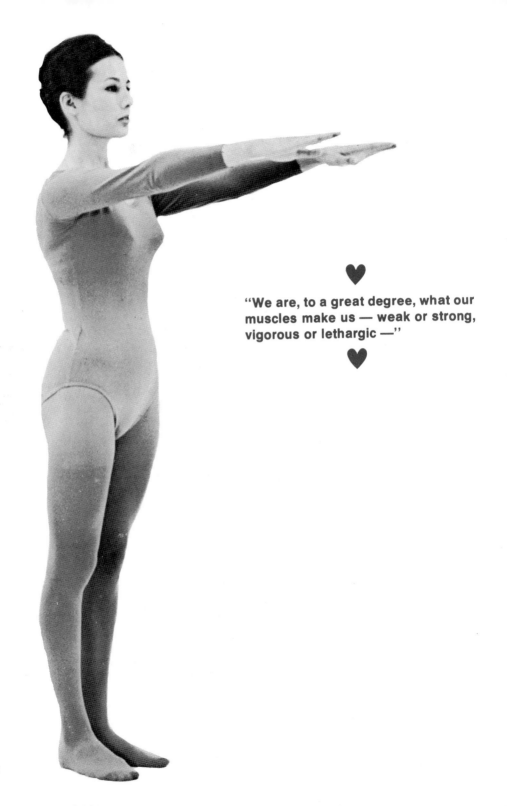

"We are, to a great degree, what our muscles make us — weak or strong, vigorous or lethargic —"

Some training tips

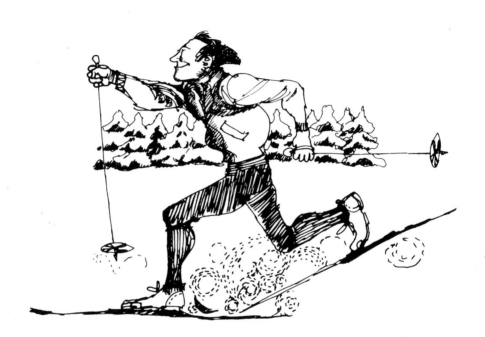

Your training goals

The goal is to devote two or three half-hour periods a week to training. The reason for this form of training is that walking and running are natural activities. With large muscle groups at work doing these actions, exertion is moderate and the training effect is still good. You are not dependent on others, as in team sports, and you can always find some place to train, even while traveling in your own country or abroad. It does not matter if you train in the morning, afternoon, or evening.

Practical circumstances will decide your schedule. Your tempo should be adapted to your degree of fitness, health, and age. It should not be extended beyond a certain level and speed should not be your objective.

The course illustrates a basic principle in all training: large muscle groups work at varying speeds. Other sports can be designed according to the same principle. Joint and muscle exercises can be done most simply at home, but for overall fitness, you need to get all your muscle groups working together.

Why speed is not important

At present, covering as long a distance as possible within 12 minutes is a popular training method. In my opinion, this is overdoing things, from a physiological point of view. As was pointed out earlier, it is not necessary to aim at maximal performance if the goal is to improve the function of the cardiovascular system and to burn extra calories. As far as health is concerned, it is not the absolute amount and volume of training that is important, but the work in relation to the individual's capacity is what is critical. The severe, prolonged training of the top athlete adds no health benefits to those of a sub-maximal training program twice a week. It would be a pity if point systems and stopwatches should become the be-all and end-all of regular physical activity.

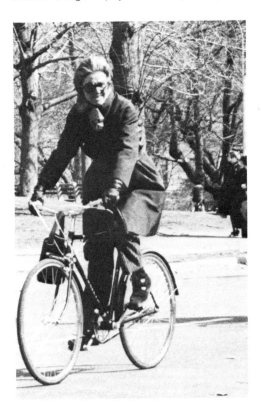

How hard a pace should be sustained?

As we mentioned previously, an effective training program should have large muscle groups working hard — but not at a maximum — for a few minutes. The reason why the pace should not be at a maximum is as follows: if you run at a certain pace (for example, seven miles per hour), the combustion engine, with its demand for oxygen transported by the blood, supplies the energy. When speed is further increased, the anaerobic motor has to satisfy the increased energy demands while the load on the heart is not further increased. The seven miles per hour speed provides full exercise for the heart and circulation while a still higher tempo develops the ability to utilize anaerobic processes and to tolerate lactic acid (the waste product of muscular activity). Training at maximum speed for a minute or so is very strenuous. It is an inevitable part of the athlete's training program, but it is wise to exclude it from an average person's training program. The conclusion is, thus, that a distance that can be covered in about three minutes can be run in three and one-half or even four minutes without being less effective in conditioning the cardiovascular function.

As a guide, I would say that if the heart rate rises to 200 minus your age in years (for example 165 for a 35-year-old), a good training effect is being achieved.

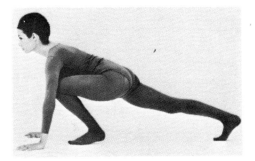

Checking your heart rate

To determine if you are exercising at the correct intensity, stop your activity momentarily, take your pulse for 10 seconds and then multiply that number of beats by 6. Check the chart following and see if your pulse rate falls within the target zone (Figure 9). In the beginning keep your pulse rate near the lower limit. As you become more fit, your target heart rate can approach the upper limit.

**Heart Rate
Target Zone**

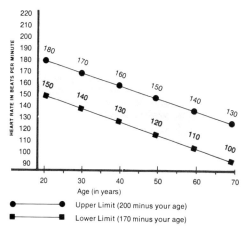

Fig. 9.

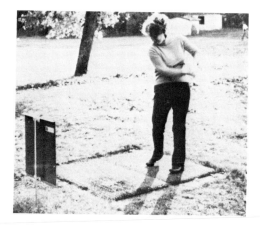

Caloric consumption

Within wide limits, when walking fast, jogging, or running, the speed is unimportant as a determinant of the energy cost per mile. The point is then to cover a certain distance. A 150- to 160-lb. person consumes about 50 Calories by walking at three miles per hour and about 80 Calories by walking at five miles per hour or running at any speed about half a mile. Taking walks, preferably a mile or so a day, will provide long-term benefits. You could, for example, get off the bus a few stops earlier and get on a few stops later. If it's not too far, you can walk or cycle to work in good weather.

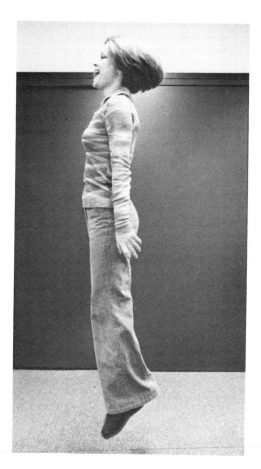

Tips for women

As you begin your training program, you should have no fear of becoming heavily, unattractively muscled. On the contrary, with disuse or little use, muscles tend to become less elastic, weaker, softer. They lose tone. The exercises you will be working with are designed to firm your muscles, restore their tone, increase their strength and flexibility. Your appearance will improve as certain muscles — in the abdomen and back, for example — become able to provide better support. As others — in the arms, legs — become more responsive, every move you make is likely to be easier and more graceful.

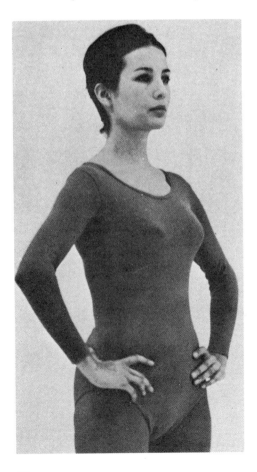

Ergometry and the ergometer

The term *ergometry* stems from the Greek *ergon* (work) and *metron* (measure), and it may be translated rather literally as "work measurement." The instruments of work measurement are ergometers, and they vary in their construction according to the form of analysis. Bicycling has proved to be a very suitable work form since, among other things, at a given (sub-maximal) load, it demands about the same energy output whether the subject is young or old, trained or out of condition, elite cyclist or unfamiliar with the sport.

The bicycle ergometer was invented several decades ago and has been widely used in physiological laboratories ever since. This instrument provides an exact measurement of the performed external work and thus a graded measureable load can be applied to the subject. The load is adjusted quite simply be varying the tension of a belt running around the rim of the one wheel of the machine, acting as a mechanical brake, while the subject pedals at a constant speed in time with a metronome.

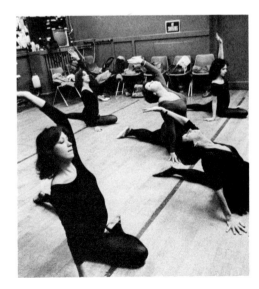

On a stationary bicycle ergometer a standard, sub-maximal work load is applied for six minutes, the heart rate being counted during the last minutes of exercise and noted. In principle the lower the heart rate, the better is the pumping power of the heart. The heart rate of an untrained subject may reach 170 beats per minute during the test. If he or she then starts to train a couple of times a week, and after a month is tested again, the heart rate may be found to have fallen to 140 beats per minute, showing that the training has been effective.

This test has proved to be a valuable educational and psychological tool for stimulating people to start and to continue training. In Sweden, there are now about 6,000 bicycle ergometers in use. They are available in every school and also in sports clubs, factories, and offices; anyone who is interested can take the sub-maximal test and follow his or her physical condition over the years.

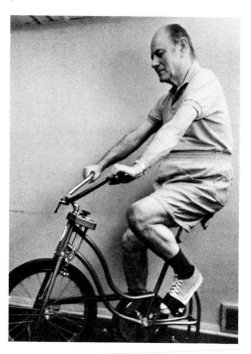

Water activities

Swimming is one of the best physical activities for people of all ages — and for many of the handicapped. With the body submerged in water, blood circulation automatically increases to some extent; pressure of water on the body also helps promote deeper ventilation of the lungs; and with well-planned activity, both circulation and ventilation increase still more.

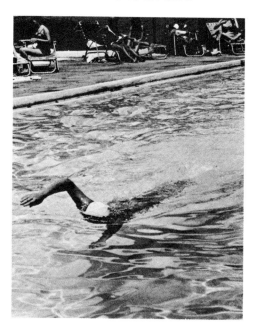

Weight training

Weight training also is an excellent method of developing muscular strength and endurance. Where equipment is available, it may be used as a supplement to conditioning exercises. Both barbells and weighted dumbbells are available at most sporting goods stores. A good rule to follow in deciding the maximum weight you should lift is to select a weight you can lift six times without strain.

Sports

Soccer, basketball, handball, squash, ice hockey, and other sports that require sustained effort can be valuable aids to building endurance. But if you have been sedentary, it is important to pace yourself carefully in such sports, and it may even be advisable to avoid them until you are well along in your physical conditioning program. That doesn't mean you should avoid all sports. Excellent sports in which exertion can be easily controlled and in which you can progress at your own rate are bicycling, hiking, skating, tennis, running, cross-country skiing, rowing, canoeing, water skiing, and skin diving. You can engage in these sports at any time in the program, if you start slowly. Games should be played with full speed and vigor only when your conditioning permits doing so without undue fatigue. For a view of sports by the experts, see the Appendix.

Posture

There is a relationship between good posture and physical fitness — one helps the other. Good posture acts to avoid cramping of internal organs, permits better circulation, prevents undue tensing of some muscles and undue lengthening of others. It contributes to fitness.

For good posture, centers of gravity of many parts of the body — feet, legs, hips, trunk, shoulders, and head — must be in a vertical line. As veiwed from the side when you are standing, the line should run through ear lobe, tip of shoulder, middle of hips, just back of kneecap, just in front of outer ankle bone. Get the feel of proper posture positions. Practice them until they become habitual.

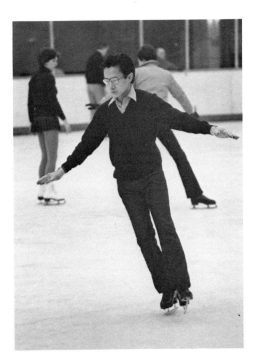

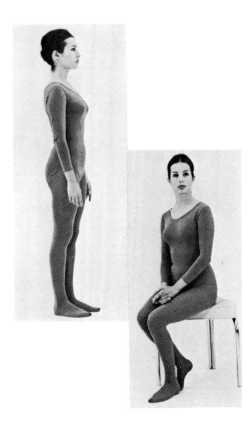

Strength training and isometric exercises

A distinction should be made between isometric or static and dynamic work. With static contraction of the muscles there is no movement in the joints in question but movement arises with dynamic work. There are in fact few exercises which are completely dynamic since a great many muscles always have to work statically to provide muscles working dynamically with good support and work conditions.

If you wish to improve your maximum strength, you must work against hard resistance. Endurance training, on the other hand, is best undertaken with lighter resistance and with many repetitions.

For general training of the muscles, work should be chosen against a load big enough to be managed just 5-10 times. You can use barbell weights, muscle developers, or your own body weight as loads. Strong persons could, for example, do 5-10 push-ups at a fast pace. Weaker persons could do the push-ups with their hands on a sofa, table, or wall instead of the floor. The position of the hands can be lowered as muscle strength increases.

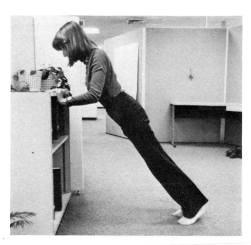

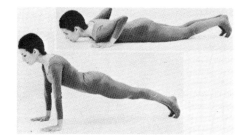

You can strengthen your abdominal muscles by lying on the floor on your back with knees bent and lifting your trunk with full sit-ups. The movement is easier if the feet are supported. It should be done 4-16 times, possibly repeated after a pause.

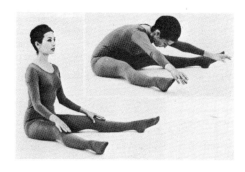

The back muscles can be forced to work if you lie on your stomach and try to lift your legs and the upper part of your trunk off the floor. People with stiff backs should lie on a proper cushion placed on a level with the pelvis (see Fig. 9). The exercise is repeated some 4 to 16 times.

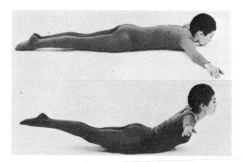

Leg muscles are trained by walking up stairs, skipping rope, and jumping or running in place. A good way to train is to climb up and down from a steady chair — the classic (but somewhat boring) step test! Running 20-25 strides up a steep hill or up as many stairs, walking down and then running up again about 5 times is also effective training in this respect.

Muscular strength is dependent on both muscle mass and the function of the central nervous system. The repetition of a given movement will result in an improvement in that particular activity, but will have much less effect on another movement, even if it happens to be related. The transfer effect, as it is called, is fairly weak. Personally, I believe that dynamic exercises have a more all-around effect than isometric training. Certainly trunk muscles work predominantly isometrically in many daily activities, but they will become trained for these tasks, for in many of the activities that engage the arms and legs they work isometrically to stabilize the pelvis and trunk.

Cardiac patients should avoid isometric exercises and also heavy work involving small muscle groups (like push-ups, chin-ups). Such activities load the heart abnormally since the heart rate and arterial blood pressure become higher than in dynamic work with large muscles.

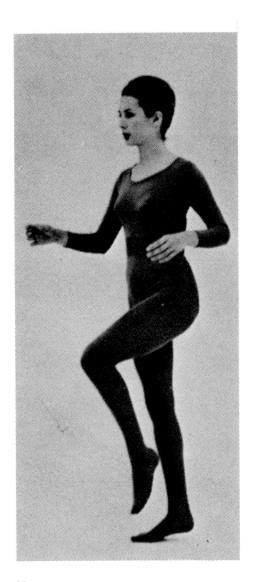

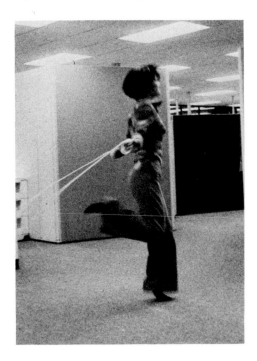

Smoking and its effects

Within a few minutes of smoking two cigarettes, a person's breathing resistance increases to two or three times the normal value. He or she may not notice this increase at rest, since relatively little air is required, but breathing may become the limiting factor during exercise with these increased demands on the respiratory system. The smoker is usually short of breath with a little exertion.

Smoking also affects the heart and blood circulation. Two cigarettes just before muscle work may, thus, raise a person's heart rate to a level 20 to 30 beats above the normal. Both the carbon monoxide and the nicotine in the smoke play important roles in triggering this increase in the heart rate. Carbon monoxide combines with the hemoglobin in the red blood cells 250 times more readily than oxygen. A smoker may have about 5% or more of his or her blood cells blocked by carbon monoxide and the presence of this gas makes it more difficult for the red blood cells to yield oxygen to the tissues. Thus, the smoker's heart has to pump more blood per unit of time in order to transport a given volume of oxygen, and the load on the heart increases. Recent evidence has shown that nicotine levels in the blood are contributory factors in disease and arteriosclerosis and coronary disease. Accordingly, smoking causes a decline in a person's physical condition, the extent of which is determined by the number of cigarettes smoked. Cigarettes, it should be mentioned, have a greater unfavorable effect on the body than cigar or pipe smoking.

The instinct of self-preservation undoubtedly explains why athletes in endurance seldom or never smoke!

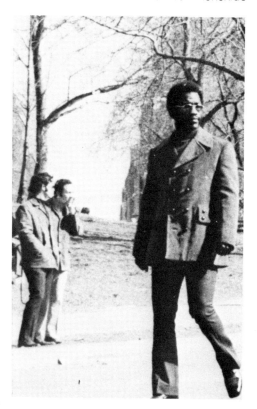

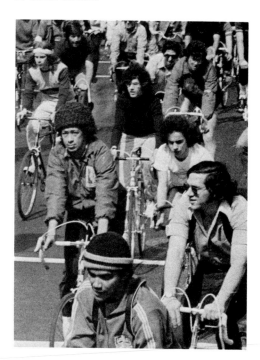

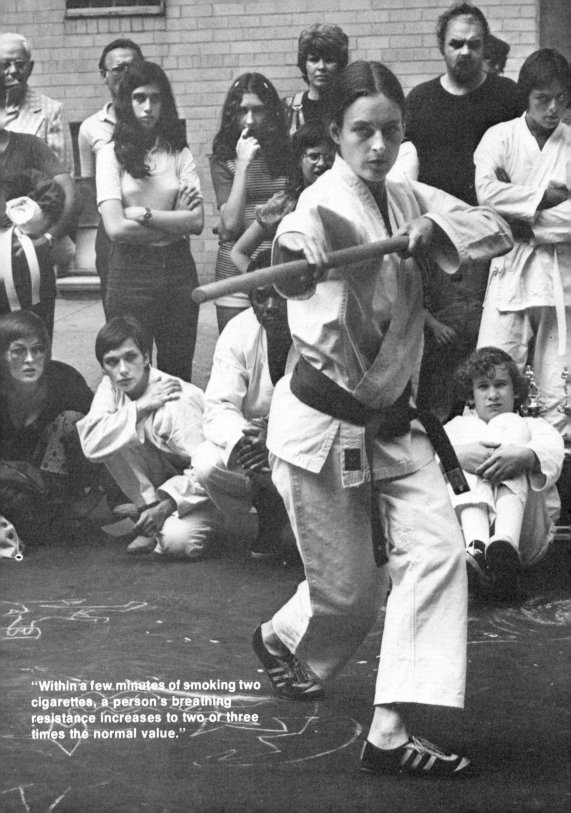

"Within a few minutes of smoking two cigarettes, a person's breathing resistance increases to two or three times the normal value."

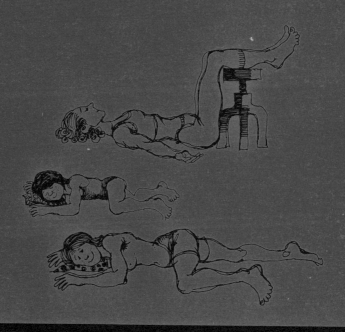

 Fitness facts

The following are the physiological responses the body makes to various degrees of exercise. Depending upon the type of activity, the body adjusts the amount of air breathed, the amount of oxygen consumed, the number of beats the heart makes, and the number of Calories it uses.

Type of activity	Respiration liters of air/min	Oxygen consumed liters/min	Heart rate beats/min	Energy expended Calories/min
At rest	10	.33	70	1.5
Very light	20	1.0	100	5.0
Light	30	1.5	110	7.5
Moderate	40	2.0	120	10.0
Heavy	60	3.0	140	15.0
Very heavy	70	3.5	150	16.5
Maximum	120	5.0	200	25.0

*Based on data obtained from college-age men of varying physical condition

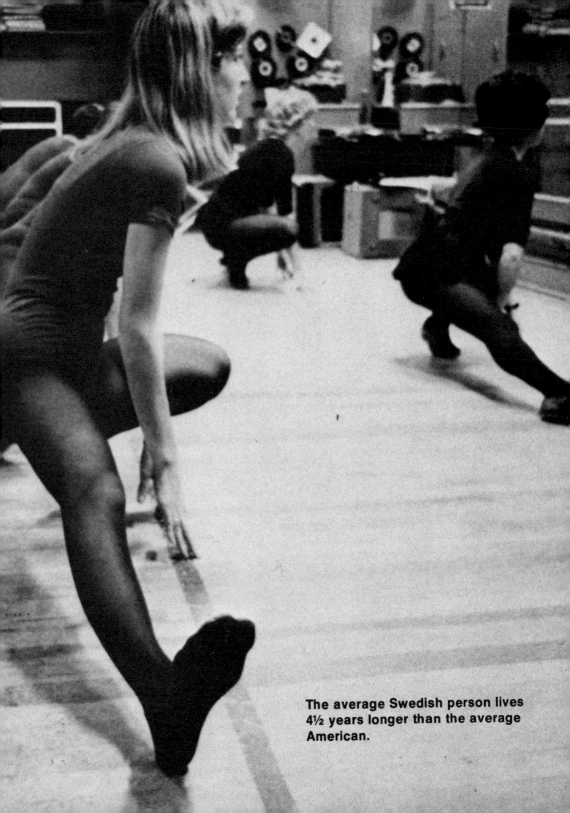

The average Swedish person lives
4½ years longer than the average
American.

Concluding remarks

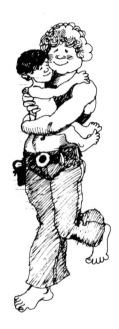

Society has a big responsibility

As pointed out in the introduction, it costs a lot of money for society to care for the sick. If sick days and poor health could be partly prevented, great savings would be achieved. The money a community invests in active recreation and training may provide tenfold dividends in money saved on medical service costs. The problem that must be faced is that the individual from puberty onward is lazy and the exercise table has to serve "goodies" which tempt people's appetite for training and active recreation. Laying out the Swedish training track,

preferably with changing rooms and steam baths (saunas), costs relatively little compared to medical service costs.

It is important to get young people interested in regular training at an early stage. Unfortunately, school curricula tend to reduce the time available for physical training and recreation rather than increase it. This is regrettable since it is during their school years that young people must acquire understanding and motivation and learn the program that is so important for good habits including continued regular exercise. Anything neglected during adolescence can in many cases not be made up for later on.

Swedish schools, like those in most countries, have in the past placed too much emphasis on advanced teaching of zoology, biochemistry, and the description of isolated organs when dealing with human biology. This has been at the expense of discussion of the function of the *intact* human body, at rest and during activity. The deeper the knowledge of these functions, the better are the chances to "service" the body properly and to manage the environment.

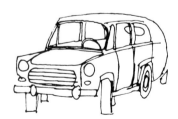

However, the Swedish schools and universities have one advantage with regard to physical education. The teaching and curriculum are almost exclusively aimed at general training and recreation. The time and resources spent on competitive sports and the coaching of athletes are very limited.

Efforts are made to provide service and education for everyone, from the handicapped to the physically fit person. Pupils and students who are endowed for and interested in competitive sports are stimulated to join any of the many sport clubs, normally independent of the schools. After finishing school it is then natural for the former student to continue his sport activities under the auspices of the sport club.

It should also be mentioned that most trade unions organize major sports programs and various outdoor activities (games, skating, bicycling, etc., often as family activities). Such activities are subsidized by the company, and the managers also participate! This sector sponsors soccer, ice hockey, handball, basketball leagues, etc., and the motivation to participate seems to follow the motto of the founder of the modern Olympic Games, Baron Pierre de Coubertin: "The important thing is to participate, not to win!"

In Swedish cities and communities, sidewalks are not only provided in the central areas, but in outlying suburbs as well. In my opinion, there has been too much emphasis on the auto while the need for safe walking space has been neglected. There should also be a strenuous program to build safe bicycling lanes and trails to supplement the main roads.

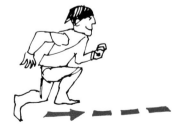

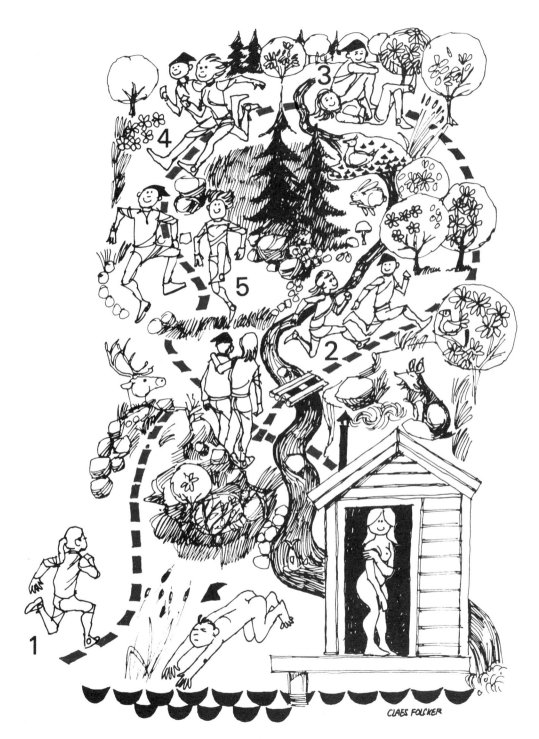

CLAES FOLCKER

Remember!

Exercise regularly, preferably two to three times a week.

Exercise at a modest tempo the first few times, increase the pace slowly, and don't "push too hard"; speed should not be maximal!

Never take part in a competition involving physical exertion when you are out of shape, no matter what kind of competition.

Don't exercise hard and don't compete when you have any infection.

Forget now and then that there are things like elevators, buses, and cars. Remember from time to time that you have legs and that there are forests and grounds for sports and open air activities.

I have heard that medical cases have been brought into the law courts with the following background: A man was advised by his physician to start an exercise program. However, he suffered a heart attack. He maintained that the exercise and, indirectly, the doctor were to blame, and therefore the doctor should bear the financial burden. Such a trial has never been and, I hope, never will be brought up in Sweden.

(It would be more logical for the habitually *inactive* person who had a heart attack to "accuse" his physician for not warning him that inactivity was a risk factor for the development of cardiovascular disease.)

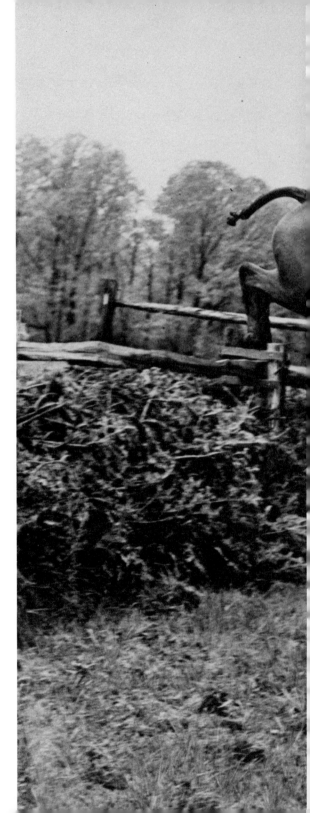

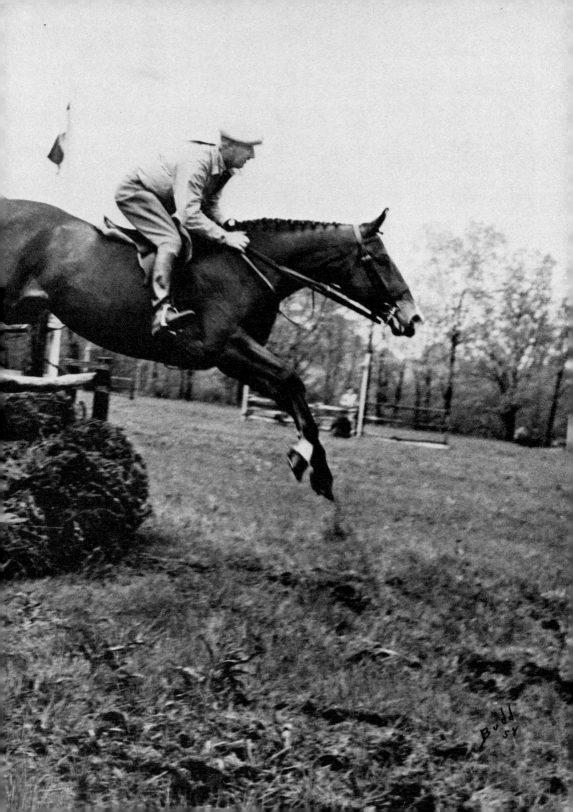

Budd '5?

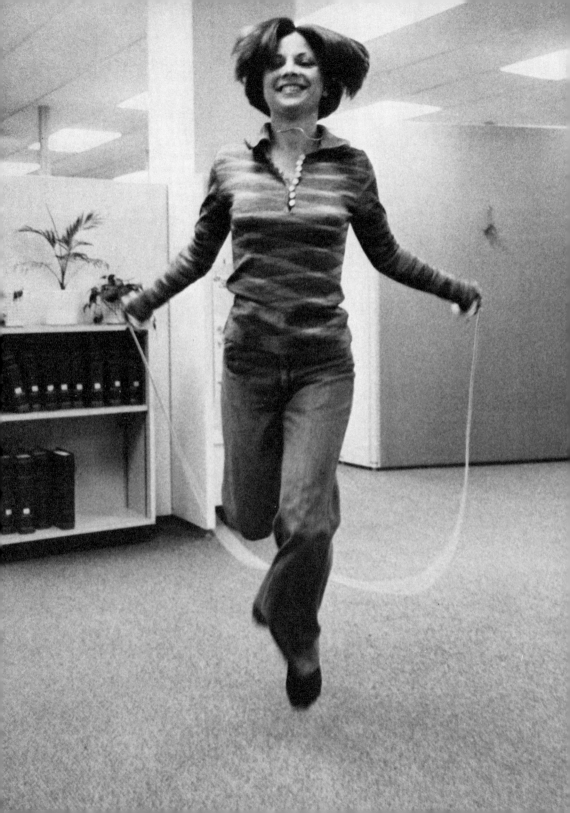

Appendix: How different sports rate in promoting physical fitness*

C. Carson Conrad
Executive Director, President's Council on
Physical Fitness and Sports

It is a well known medical fact that when a person is immobilized for long periods of time or confined to bed, the bones lose their calcium, the kidneys and bowels lose their functional efficiency, the somatic muscles rapidly become weak and flabby, and the heart and circulation lose their tone and ability to respond to even the slightest stress. One of the most striking medical findings of the 11 Apollo moon missions was the revelation of the extent and rapidity with which these degenerative changes developed in space, where confinement and lack of gravity reduced exercise to a minimum. In this and in many other studies it was clearly demonstrated that use and exercise are necessary to maintain the functional integrity of various body systems.

But what kind of use and what kind of exercise will best promote the highest level of efficiency of the body? Our panel of seven medical experts selected 14 popular but diverse forms of exercise for evaluation in terms of their special contributions to physical well being. Some of these, such as basketball and tennis, can be regarded as "sports"; others, such as calisthenics, walking and jogging, are more commonly looked upon as merely popular forms of exercise. The evaluation of the 14 different forms of exercise was made in terms of regular participation (a minimum of four times a week) and vigorous activity (a duration of not less than a half hour).

Initially the experts also were asked to consider the different exercises from the standpoint of their influence on sexual performance. This was eliminated from the present summation because the experts considered no one sport to be inherently more "sexy" than the others. Furthermore, it was generally agreed that good physical condition from any kind of exercise undoubtedly has a beneficial effect on this as well as other functions of the human body.

*This article is reprinted from *Medical Times*, May 1976. Reprinted by permission.

A quick rating of 14 sports and/or exercises is shown in the "Scorecard" on the next spread. Following are specific comments by our panel of exercise experts.

Jogging

Fox: The most efficient and inexpensive approach to enhancing endurance capacity. Must be approached with warm-up preliminaries and a "starter" program of walk-jog alternations.

Lamb: This is an endurance exercise that will not build muscle mass beyond the natural size of the body. Running faster and faster is not a great advantage. It takes almost the same amount of energy (calories) to run one and a half miles in sixteen minutes as it does to run it in eight minutes. I estimate an average of 720 calories per hour.

Ryan: A great activity to promote fitness. The results come slowly, however.

Kraus: Excellent for cardiovascular fitness; unfit people should start with a calisthenics program first to attain minimum muscular fitness, otherwise muscle strain, back pain, etc., often result.

Gendel: Excellent "all around" activity—especially the ability to begin in stages at any age—therefore beneficial to body systems—even those that have been

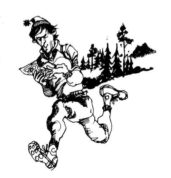

subject to debilitating disease and need rehabilitation.

Guild: Plus—can squeeze a maximum consistent effort into a minimum amount of time. Minus—can be boring.

Klumpp: One can adjust the pace and distance to one's own particular condition and fitness.

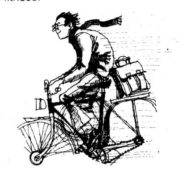

Bicycling

Kraus: Good fitness-building activity, primarily cardiovascular. Calorie consuming.

Klumpp: Bicycling with the pedal at the instep fails to give maximum extension to the ankle and foot. It is important to adjust the seat so that the leg is fully extended when the pedal is at the bottom of the circle.

Ryan: A great fitness activity when indulged in regularly at a good steady pace.

Guild: Plus—good for endurance and can be done alone (thus no need to program this into other people's schedules). Minus—ice, snow, fog (rain is okay).

Gendel: A "forever" activity in health and fitness. It rates high for development of leg and back muscle strength.

Fox: Excellent if vigorously pursued. Good endurance-generating exercise.

Lamb: An endurance exercise—estimate 400 calories an hour—depending upon speed and road conditions.

Swimming

Guild: Plus—good for total body conditioning; a nonweight-bearing sport, it's good for people recovering from hip, knee, and ankle problems. Minus—requires availability of a pool.

Fox: Excellent as endurance-stimulator and for total body development. Is important that all citizens be comfortable in the water to avoid high incidence of drowning deaths—must be a part of school curriculum requirements.

Klumpp: Magnificent exercise, but it neglects the weight-bearing, antigravity musculature of the body and should be balanced by something like jogging for ideal, all-around muscular development.

Gendel: One of the excellent, all-around physical activities.

Ryan: Excellent for fitness. As good as running if you can swim well enough.

Kraus: Excellent for fitness maintenance and for cardiovascular fitness.

Lamb: Primarily an endurance exercise; depends on speed and stroke used; estimate 500 calories per hour on the average.

Ice/roller skating

Gendel: Most people don't indulge in these sports unless they do them well, which means they learned them early in life; excellent sports once learned and used.

Klumpp: Skating does a lot for the pelvis and legs; for ideal all-round development, it should be supplemented with upper body exercise.

Fox: Good endurance effects with delightful social attributes at modest cost; satisfying skill and agility aspects.

Kraus: Good for fitness building and maintenance for people who have the necessary muscular fitness.

Ryan: Both are great for fitness when done on a vigorous basis.

Guild: Plus—good for endurance and agility. Minus—not enough indoor and outdoor rinks.

Lamb: Estimate 640 calories an hour. Primarily an endurance exercise.

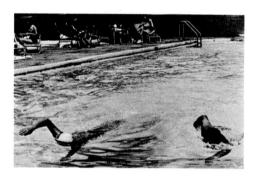

Handball/squash

Klumpp: When vigorously played, provides a maximum of exercise in a minimum of time.

Fox: Excellent endurance stimulation. Should warm up prior to play. Demands of ligaments and joints may cause problems in middle to later years.

Kraus: Good fitness maintaining sport if played regularly by fit people.

Gendel: Excellent on almost all counts because of the agility it promotes.

Guild: Plus—good for endurance and agility. Minus—there aren't enough courts.

Lamb: Vigorous endurance-type exercise; estimate 1000 calories per hour.

Ryan: Largely anaerobic activity. Will keep you fit if played on a regular basis, however.

A quick scorecard on 14 sports and exercises

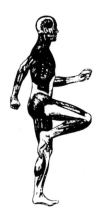

Here's a summary of how the seven experts quoted in this article rated the various sports and exercises discussed. Ratings are on a scale of 0 to 3, thus a rating of 21 indicates maximum benefit (a score of 3 by all 7 panelists). Ratings were made on the basis of regular (minimum of 4 times per week), vigorous (duration of 30 minutes to one hour per session) participation in each activity.

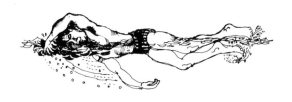

		Jogging	Bicycling	Swimming	Skating (Ice or Roller)	Handball Squash
Physical fitness	Cardiorespiratory endurance (stamina)	21	19	21	18	19
	Muscular endurance	20	18	20	17	18
	Muscular strength	17	16	14	15	15
	Flexibility	9	9	15	13	16
	Balance	17	18	12	20	17
General well-being	Weight control	21	20	15	17	19
	Muscle definition	14	15	14	14	11
	Digestion	13	12	13	11	13
	Sleep	16	15	16	15	12
	Total	148	142	140	140	140

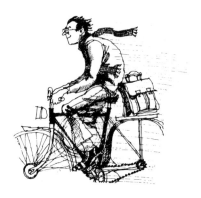

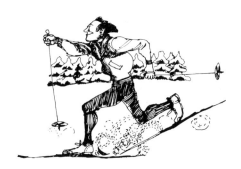

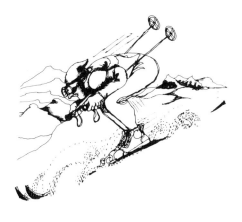
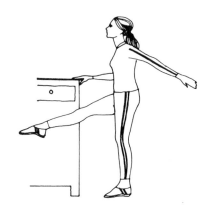

Skiing-Nordic	Skiing-Alpine	Basketball	Tennis	Calisthenics	Walking	Golf*	Softball	Bowling
19	16	19	16	10	13	8	6	5
19	18	17	16	13	14	8	8	5
15	15	15	14	16	11	9	7	5
14	14	13	14	19	7	8	9	7
16	21	16	16	15	8	8	7	6
17	15	19	16	12	13	6	7	5
12	14	13	13	18	11	6	5	5
12	9	10	12	11	11	7	8	7
15	12	12	11	12	14	6	7	6
139	134	134	128	126	102	66*	64	51

*Ratings for golf are based on the fact that many Americans use a golf cart and/or caddy. If you walk the links, the physical fitness value moves up appreciably. See comments of individual panelists.

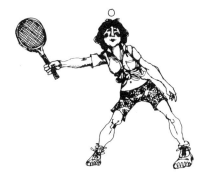
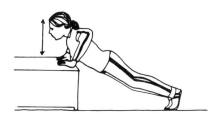

Alpine skiing—downhill and slalom
Nordic skiing—cross country and jumping

Lamb: Alpine—mostly an endurance exercise, estimate 540 calories per hour. Nordic—also an endurance exercise, but uses more calories; estimate close to 1000 per hour.

Kraus: Alpine—can maintain and improve fitness. It is especially important to have good basic muscular fitness, otherwise there is great exposure to injury. Nordic—excellent for fitness; need to be preconditioned to gain maximum muscular fitness.

Fox: Alpine—some endurance stimulating value; excellent for leg and back development. Nordic—excellent endurance-stimulating activity with good arm-shoulder development.

Klumpp: Both are excellent sports and offer the additional advantage of the metabolic stimulation provided by low temperatures.

Guild: Alpine—plus—good for agility; minus—expensive. Nordic—plus—good for endurance; minus—requires equipment and, usually, travel time.

Gendel: Alpine—except for the high risk factor for injury, this can be excellent. Nordic—long term carry-over activity.

Ryan: Alpine—does little for fitness but you must be fit to avoid injury. Nordic—a great sport to promote endurance.

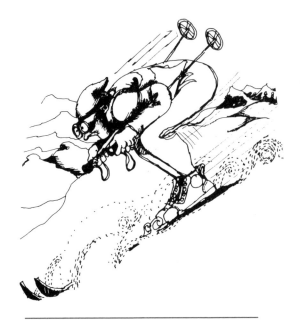

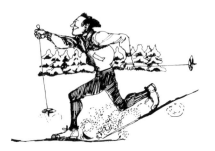

Basketball

Ryan: A sport for the already fit. You don't play basketball to *get* fit; you must *be* fit to play it.

Guild: Plus—good for endurance and agility. Minus—try to find ten guys four times a week!

Lamb: Uses lots of energy, about 1000 calories per hour for the average adult.

Kraus: Good fitness-maintaining sport if played regularly by fit people.

Gendel: Obviously contributes to general fitness and health, but because of its team nature, it may or may not lead to ongoing, carryover "life" activities.

Klumpp: From a physical fitness standpoint, an excellent sport.

Fox: Excellent endurance-generating exercise with great stimulus for enhancing coordination, agility. Good for school/college years. Moderate hazards of injury and strain on joints and ligaments may discourage post-collegiate involvement.

Tennis

Ryan: If you run for the balls, it's a great game to keep you fit.

Gendel: An excellent all-around activity which may carry some of the same anxiety levels inherent in golf and other sports where people worry about their game.

Klumpp: Splendid exercise for almost all purposes except bilateral symmetrical upper-body development; its value for the development of cardiovascular fitness depends on the manner in which one plays.

Fox: Excellent for body shaping, flexibility and balance; stimulates endurance if vigorously played.

Lamb: Moderate endurance exercise—estimate 500 calories an hour.

Kraus: Good for cardiovascular fitness and muscular fitness.

Guild: Plus—good for endurance and agility. Minus—seasonal, not enough indoor courts.

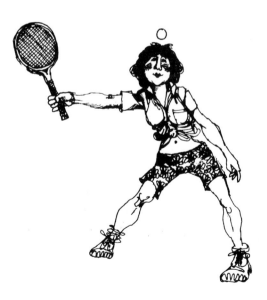

The seven experts on physical fitness

Samuel M. Fox III, M.D.
Professor of Medicine, Georgetown University; Former President, American College of Cardiology; Former Chief, Heart Disease Control Program, USPHS

Evalyn S. Gendel, M.D.
Assistant Director, Bureau of Maternal & Child Health, Kansas State Department of Health and Environment; and Adjunct Professor, Department of Human Ecology and Community Health, Kansas University Medical School

Warren R. Guild, M.D.
Past President of The American College of Sports Medicine; Clinical Associate in Medicine, Harvard Medical School

Theodore G. Klumpp, M.D.
Medical Consultant to The President's Council on Physical Fitness and Sports

Hans Kraus, M.D.
Clinical Associate Professor of Physical Medicine and Rehabilitation, New York University Medical School, and co-developer of the Kraus-Weber Test for strength and flexibility.

Lawrence E. Lamb, M.D.
Former Professor of Medicine, Baylor Medical School; Former Chief of Cardiology, Sheppard Air Force Base Hospital; Syndicated medical columnist

Allan J. Ryan, M.D.
Professor of Physical Education and Rehabilitation Medicine, University of Wisconsin

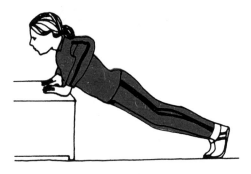

Calisthenics

Kraus: A good calisthenics program should contain relaxation and limbering exercises, should build up slowly from relaxation to warm-up to workout and then return to cool-off and finally relaxation.

Fox: Flexibility enhancement, very useful for most ages. Endurance stimulation may not be great unless rigorously pursued.

Klumpp: Its value rests entirely on the vigor of the exercise program; properly prescribed exercises are particularly valuable for muscle and joint flexibility and back problems.

Guild: Plus—good for total body conditioning if done for strength and stamina and not for muscle hypertrophy. Minus—boring as hell!!

Lamb: Can develop muscle mass and can be both endurance and strength type exercise.

Ryan: When these are scheduled in a circuit training program they promote physical fitness very well.

Gendel: Can be done alone, in pairs, in groups, and can involve music and experimentation with body mechanics.

Walking

Fox: Excellent for reconditioning, but not a great added stimulus for those in "good" condition.

Klumpp: Excellent if one has time to walk far enough, fast enough. Ideal for the lame, blind, halt, and decrepit!

Kraus: Excellent. But requires more time and faster walking to attain cardiovascular fitness.

Ryan: Great for fitness if done at a brisk, steady pace.

Gendel: Excellent exercise because anyone can do it—alone, in pairs, in groups, etc. Can be graduated in intensity for any age or physical limitation.

Guild: Plus—good for endurance, especially when combined with normal, daily activities. Minus—takes a lot of time unless pace is brisk.

Lamb: Moderate endurance exercise—estimate 250 calories an hour.

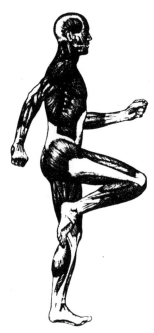

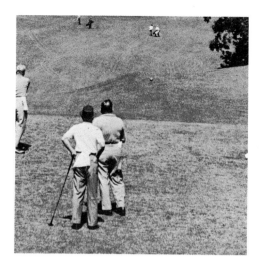

Golf

Klumpp: A fine recreational pastime, but as played today utilizing a caddy and/or a golf cart, it provides so little exercise that it is practically useless from the physical-fitness standpoint.

Ryan: Does little or nothing for fitness unless you walk and carry your clubs or play on a hilly course.

Kraus: Little fitness value.

Guild: Plus—good for relaxation and camaraderie. Minus—little physiological benefit . . . and it's expensive.

Gendel: The large social and club element associated with it often offsets its ability to accomplish positive points. Continual "fretting" about one's game does not help digestion or sleep.

Lamb: An endurance-type exercise; uses about 300 calories per hour.

Fox: If walking and carrying bag of clubs, golf has moderate stimulus for aerobic endurance for those of only moderate or less fitness, but caddies and electric carts lessen these aspects.

Softball

Guild: Plus—few injuries; good for agility. Minus—too much time sitting around doing nothing.

Klumpp: Good fun. Excellent recreation, but too little exercise.

Kraus: No good to create fitness; not too valuable for fitness maintenance either.

Ryan: Does little or nothing for fitness.

Lamb: Moderate exercise; estimate 280 calories per hour, except for pitcher who may use an additional 100 calories.

Fox: Pleasant activity with skill and agility benefits.

Gendel: Depends, once again, on involvement in the activity, and may or may not have life-long value.

Bowling

Fox: A pleasant recreation but not useful in enhancing fitness. May eat and drink more calories than activity burns up.

Ryan: Does nothing to promote physical fitness—just a good game.

Klumpp: Not enough exercise to have a pronounced effect on physical fitness, but it's better than nothing.

Lamb: The lightest exercise in the group. Estimate only 150 calories an hour. It won't do as much for you as a good walk.

Kraus: Little fitness value.

Gendel: It's social nature for the general public is associated with opportunities for food intake (and beverages).

Guild: Plus—good for recreation, skill and camaraderie. Minus—no significant physiological benefits.

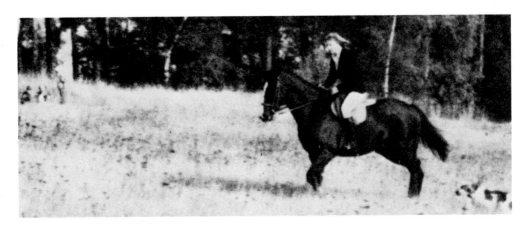

Some opinions on other sports and exercises

About volleyball, canoeing, water-skiing, and horseback riding, Dr. Fox says:

"Volleyball is less demanding than basketball and can be easier to organize teams with odd numbers and less equal skills than with basketball. A good mix of exertion and sociability.

"Canoeing is good total body exercise if done vigorously as in stream or whitewater padding (with associated hazards).

"Water-skiing is good fun but noisy, and needs expensive equipment. Largely isometric, with anxiety component which makes it not good for heart disease patients.

"Horseback riding provides good exercise but is expensive and there is some hazard."

Dr. Lamb points out that ". . . unless they are included in calisthenics, we have omitted real strength-type exercises, such as muscle training or weight training, from our consideration. That is a mistake because developing good strong muscles is part of maintaining good posture, which is important to health as well as appearance."

About team sports, Dr. Kraus says: "For school-years fitness, team sports and any other sports should come second to fitness-creating activities which include jogging, running, and calisthenics for basic minimum muscular fitness. Team sports are most likely to back-fire and give only the most fit a chance to compete, leaving on the sidelines the ones who need activity the most."

And Dr. Gendel points out that "fitness activities of a team or group often cannot be guaranteed to continue throughout life. Also, sometimes anxiety issues related to team activities cause digestive, nervous or distractive influences affecting sleep, etc."

Dr. Gendel also regretted that the panel had not considered dancing and gymnastics: "Since fitness and sports concerns both sexes, I was sorry to see dancing (modern, ballet, folk and free form) plus gymnastics omitted from the list. These activities offer a great deal of exertion for both men and women. Their benefits are again universal for activity, alone or in groups, and also add the element of music for its psychological as well as physical input."

General summary

Including their comments, Dr. Klumpp and Dr. Lamb pointed out that, in each one of the sports listed, there is an x ingredient. This ingredient is *the way one engages in the sport or exercise.* Dr. Klumpp said "I used to bowl with a friend who stood almost motionless and gently waved the ball toward the pins, and they usually all gently fell over; whereas I would get to the back of the alley, rush to the line, and hurl the ball with as much vigor as I could muster—and I could never beat my friend. He got the scores, but I got the exercise.

"In tennis, I have friends who consider it a waste of energy to run for the ball on the theory that, even if you get it, you are so out of position that your opponent can put it away. I have never seen such players in much of a sweat or out of breath. I go for everything, and surprisingly often, even a poor return is flubbed by the opposition. Here again the calories expended and the cardiovascular stimulation depend on how one plays the game."

A general principle of great importance, in Dr. Klumpp's opinion, is the necessity of bringing about stress in exercise programs, if one engages in exercise to maintain or improve body and cardiovascular fitness. Many who do not understand biophysiology regard stress as something to be avoided. They are partially right if one thinks of extremes of stress, but in all human endeavors an insufficient amount is worthless and too much is harmful. "This is true of almost everything," says Dr. Klumpp.

He also feels that proper exercise is beneficial for an individual's physiological well-being, including digestion, sexual performance, and sleep. Dr. Lamb disagreed to some extent when he said:

"Other than its effects on building muscle mass — which may have some relation to amounts of male hormone produced — exercise has little or no effect on sex, except for weight control and prevention of atherosclerosis — which may affect the testicle. Fatty deposits in the arteries to the testicle leads to an early decline in its function. Nor do I think that exercise has much to do with digestion. And its relaxation effects are its primary value in sleep."

Dr. Kraus stressed that minimum muscular fitness is a precondition for all sports—to avoid injury—and that the inclusion of limbering exercises is essential.

Lastly, and perhaps most important, Dr. Guild, who is past president of the American College of Sports Medicine, pointed out that "time is of the essence. After all, how much time can a busy person reasonably expect to allot to physical fitness?

"A) None—if he has no interest ('I'm too busy, but when I find time . . .')—forget it.

"B) A minimum of 30 minutes 4-5 times a week is ideal — and not unreasonable — because maximal benefits toward endurance or stamina are "promoters" of cardiovascular reserve. There are 4 S's in sports — speed, skill, strength, and stamina. The first are of interest to the young. The last (stamina) adds to longevity, to vigor, to joie de vivre, to one's ability to do a day's work effectively and yet to have enough pep left over to enjoy leisure time."

References

Åstrand, P.O. and K. Rodahl. *Textbook of Work Physiology*. New York: McGraw-Hill, 1977.

Fox, S.M., J.P. Naugthon and W.L. Haskell. "Physical Activity and the Prevention of Coronary Heart Disease." *Annals of Clinical Research* 3: 404, 1971.

Morris, J.N. and M.D. Crawford. "Coronary Heart Disease and Physical Activity of Work: Evidence of a National Necropsy Survey." *British Medical Journal* 2: 1485, 1958.

Wilmore, J.H. (ed.). *Exercise and Sport Sciences Reviews*. New York: Academic Press, Inc., 1973.

White, P.D. *My Life and Medicine*. Boston: Gambit, Inc., 1971.

Photographic credits

The sources for the illustrations in this book appear below.

De Wys Inc., Cal Hulstein, *18, 19*
Image Bank, DiGiacomo, *61*
Magnum Photos, Inc., Gilles Peress, *50, 62*
Mussler, Joel, *20, 21. 27, 30, 34, 35, 38, 40, 51, 54, 55, 56, 57, 60, 61, 64, 67, 68, 69, 70, 78, 83, (r) 84, (l) 85, (l) 86, (l) 87, (r) 88, 92, 94*
Ralph F. Petersen, *96*
Photo Researchers, Inc., Bonnie Freer, *16*
Photo Researchers, Inc., Rhoda Galyn, *12, 13, 72, 82, 89*
Photo Researchers, Inc., Peter Miller, *22*
Photo Researchers, Inc., Sherry Suris, *90*
Photo Researchers, Inc., Katrina Thomas, *14, 15, 89*
President's Council on Physical Fitness and Sports, Courtesy of The, *31, 32, (top) 52, 80, (l) 84, (r) 85, (r) 86, (r) 87, (l) 88, 112*
Roberts, H. Armstrong, *74, 75, front cover*

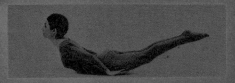

 # Fit tips

For some quick relaxation:

Loosen your clothing, take off your shoes

Stretch, lift your arms and try to touch the ceiling with your fingertips

Walk or lightly jog in place for a few minutes

Shake your shoulders and bend from your waist, first in front and then to each side

Bend your knees and touch the floor

Take a deep breath, relax

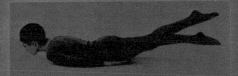